# The
# MODEL'S
# Handbook

For Every Woman Who Wants to Be
a Model or Look Like One

# The MODEL'S Handbook

### For Every Woman Who Wants to Be a Model or Look Like One

Kyle Roderick

WILLIAM MORROW AND COMPANY, INC.
New York

Library of Congress Catalog Card Number: 84-61567

ISBN 0-688-04297-X

This book was designed and produced by
Quarto Publishing Limited
32 Kingly Court, London W1

*Art Director:* Alastair Campbell
*Editorial Director:* Christopher Fagg
*Editor:* Emma Johnson
*Designer:* Jeroo Roy
*Illustrator:* Terry Evans
*Picture Research:* Keith Bernstein
*Special thanks to:* Joanna Swindell, Chris Thomson,
Elenka Zaboynikova

Typeset by QV Typesetting Limited, London
Color origination by Hong Kong Graphic Arts Service Center,
Hong Kong
Printed in Hong Kong by Lee Fung Asco Limited

First US Edition

1 2 3 4 5 6 7 8 9 10

*ACKNOWLEDGEMENTS*

*I owe thanks to the following
professionals who assisted me in the
research and writing of this book.
They are: Naomi Black, Sam Canyon,
Randy Davis, Patrick Dennis,
Jonathan Elias, Scott Elias, Nikki Gentile,
Beth Hanson, John Hoffman,
Zazel Loven, Carol Meyers, Lyne Pedola,
Shirley Krueger-Roderick,
Beth Rubino, Susan Shilling, Anne Soorikian,
and Michael Montes.*

# CONTENTS

# 4. THE MODELING WORLD

# 5. TRAVELING IN STYLE

# INTRODUCTION

Achieving goals and developing self-awareness, fitness and professionalism play an important part in every woman's personal and working life. The aim of this book is to provide sensible and effective solutions to improving your way of life, your health and your appearance — from the inside out.

*The Model's Handbook* is an essential guide for both the aspiring model and any woman who wants to look and feel her best. Not everyone can be — or wants to be — a professional model, but contained in this book are hints and inside information from full-time professionals in the beauty business which go beyond the catwalk or the photographic studio.

Beginning with fully illustrated exercise programs, diet plans and guidelines to help you organize your body care routine, you will learn how and where to start on the road to good health and beauty. Easy-to-follow make-up and hair styling methods for complementing specific face shapes, complexions and hair textures are designed to teach you how to put your best face forward. Advice from top models, model agencies, photographers and make-up artists provides you with a useful insight into the practical side of sophisticated fashion and beauty techniques.

A separate section deals with the question of whether you have what it takes to become a professional model. Are you photogenic? Do you come across well at an interview? Are you dedicated, and can you handle long photographic sessions? Practical advice is also offered on how to compile a portfolio and find a good agency to represent you. The final chapter covers travel — packing a portable beauty kit, exercising in your hotel room, how to outwit jetlag and assorted hints on how to look and feel your best when you're away.

The value of maintaining your looks, no matter what your age, cannot be emphasized enough, and the personal care programmes outlined in this book will help you reap lasting beauty and health benefits. A commitment to caring for yourself will reward you with renewed confidence and the enjoyment of worthy goals. It is never too late to change and improve if you sincerely want to. Good luck!

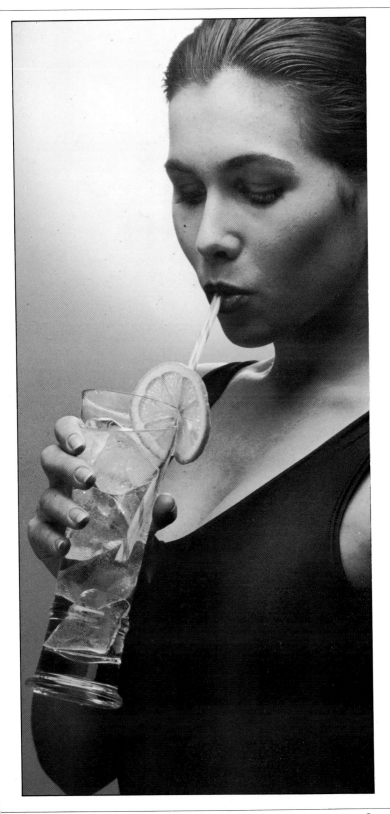

# 1
# FEELING GOOD

## KEEPING FIT

## HEALTHY EATING

*W*hen you look at yourself in a full-length mirror, does your body appear to be in good shape or is it showing the effects of erratic eating, tension, late nights and lack of exercise? Consider how your state of health is reflected in your outward appearance — your complexion, hair, eyes and figure as well as your level of energy. Feeling good is the essential key to looking good, and vice versa, and you can't achieve one state without the other. Therefore the first beauty secret to remember is that good looks are dependent upon a healthy lifestyle and general well-being.

# KEEPING FIT

Begin by evaluating your living habits: diet, sleep, exercise, skin and hair care. What is there too much of, or too little of, in your life? Do you exercise regularly, or not at all? Is your diet balanced or lacking in the essential ingredients, such as iron, vitamins, protein or roughage? Do you carefully cleanse, tone and moisturize your face according to its needs, or do you use soap and water all year round? Do you sleep less, or more than you need to? Your answers to these questions will give you a clear indication of what you should do to change or improve your lifestyle.

The first step is to make a commitment to frequent exercise. Working-out will improve almost every aspect of your health and appearance and, most importantly, will make you feel good. A well-structured exercise program will be beneficial to your body in many different ways — it will firm up flabby areas, decrease your appetite, reduce stress, increase muscle tone and give you a clear,

*There are many dance and exercise classes that you can choose from: aerobic dance, modern, jazz and ballet — all give your muscles and cardiovascular system an excellent work-out. If you're out of shape, start by taking beginner's classes to improve your fitness level and then go on to intermediate or advanced classes. Other exercise options worth considering are yoga, gymnastics and the martial arts, as they also get your body into marvellous shape.*

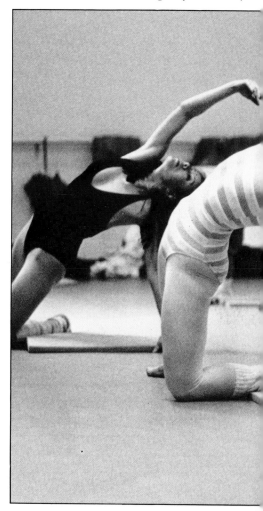

rosy complexion, better posture and more efficient circulation. The extra blood that a good workout pumps to the thyroid gland can cause it to produce more hormones that speed up the rate at which your body burns off calories. This change in your metabolism makes the digestion of food easier for your body, while also reducing the amount of sleep you need each night.

Regular exercise can be a great boon to your mental health, too. It can combat depression by increasing the flow of oxygen to the brain. It can also lengthen your attention span and make you more alert, and less susceptible to emotional upset, tension and strain. If you commit yourself to an exercise program, then your reward will be a strong and supple physique, glowing skin, improved health, and a mind that is finely tuned. Perhaps you are 35, slightly overweight, and your joints are stiff from lack of use. Now is definitely the time to correct these conditions and shape a stronger, more flexible body for yourself. Even if you are 19, skinny, and have a terrific body, there is still no excuse for you not to exercise. Get the most out of your looks and health by making your body earn its food and rest. With regular workouts, you will have more energy to enjoy life.

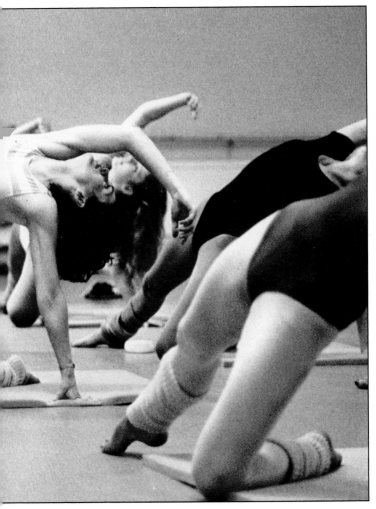

## Warm-up exercises.

Before any physical exertion, you must prepare your muscles and joints by warming them up with gentle exercises. Here are four simple warm-ups you can try. They will develop suppleness and help build muscle tone.

*1. Stand with feet 6in (15cm) apart, arms at your sides. Slowly stretch your arms out sideways, letting your wrists go limp. Flap your arms up and down rapidly, counting to 10 as you do so. Repeat several times.*

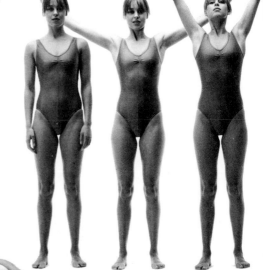

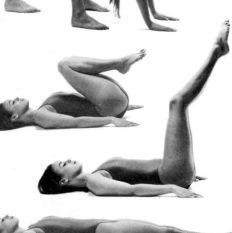

*2. Stand with legs 2ft (61cm) apart, arms at your sides. Bend forward from the waist, holding your buttocks in and stretching your palms down to the floor, as far as you can without straining. Hold for 10 seconds. In time you'll be able to hold for longer periods.*

*3. Lie flat on your back with your arms at your sides, palms on the floor. Bring both knees together up to your chest, then straighten them slowly and lower them to the floor. Repeat 10 times. This will help trim your waistline and flatten your stomach.*

*4. Wearing running shoes, run very slowly on the spot for one minute. Increase your speed, and jog for another minute.*

### Basic fitness routines

1. Lie flat on your back. Lift your head off the floor and clasp your hands behind your head. Lift your legs until they are at right angles to your body, with toes pointing inwards. Leading with your heels, spread your legs to the sides in a wide 'V' (don't allow them to fall forward or backward). When you have stretched them as far as you can, turn your heels inwards and bring them together. Repeat 10 times.

▼

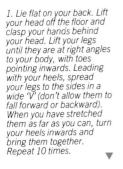

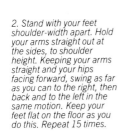

2. Stand with your feet shoulder-width apart. Hold your arms straight out at the sides, to shoulder height. Keeping your arms straight and your hips facing forward, swing as far as you can to the right, then back and to the left in the same motion. Keep your feet flat on the floor as you do this. Repeat 15 times.

▶

◀ 3. Stand with feet wide apart. Bend down to touch the floor beside your feet. Hold your head and body still, place your fists under your arms and then straighten your arms upwards. Now push them forward as far as they will go. Repeat 10 times, reversing the sequence.

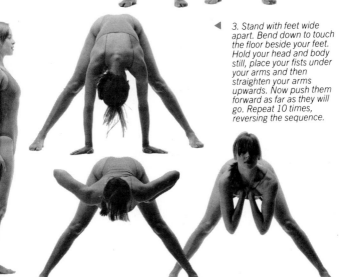

4. Stand with feet together, arms by your sides. Raise one knee as high as you can and grasp it with both hands, pulling it towards you. Hold for a few seconds and do the same with the other knee. Hold your back and head straight as you do this. Repeat 10 times. ▶

5. To perform a basic shoulder roll, stand with feet apart, arms by your sides. Shrug your shoulders up to your ears, then bring them backwards and down. Reverse the action in a rolling movement. ▼

6. Stand in front of some stairs, a sturdy low bench or a stool. Step up and back from floor to step or object in this progression: left foot up, right foot up, left foot down, right foot down. Start slowly and then gradually increase your speed. To begin with, you should do this for one minute, and work up your time and speed each day until you can do it for five minutes or more. This exercise is much more strenuous than it seems.
▼

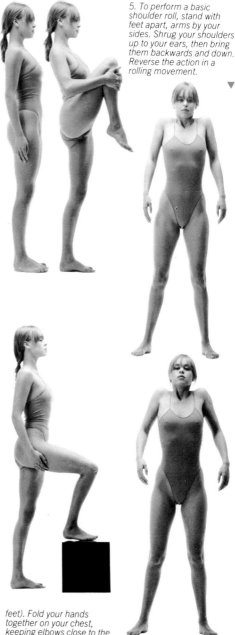

7. Sit on the floor with your back straight and knees bent. Place your feet under a firm, stationary object (or get someone to hold your ▼

feet). Fold your hands together on your chest, keeping elbows close to the body. With your back perfectly straight, lower the upper part of your body halfway to the floor and smoothly raise yourself to your original position. Repeat 10 times. Concentrate on using your stomach muscles rather than your back muscles for this exercise.

**After practising these exercises** daily for one month, you should have built up enough strength in your muscles to do twice as many without straining. If you work-out consistently in this way, your body will firm up rapidly.

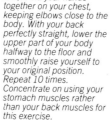

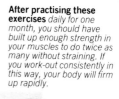

**Practical exercises for busy women**

1. Find a large, thick book or block to stand on. Place it a few inches away from a surface on which you can place your hands. Stand on this large object with the balls of your feet only and the first few inches of your instep; your heels should hang off the back. Let your heels drop down as far as they can go, and stand up on the balls of your feet, holding this position for two seconds. Although your calves will feel strained, you must maintain a slow and smooth pace to perform this exercise correctly. Repeat 15 times.

2. Lie on your right side with your right arm supporting your head. Place your left hand on the floor near your chest to balance yourself. Hold your left leg straight out, raise it as high as you can and lower it to the floor swiftly. Repeat 15 times. Turn over and repeat 15 times with the right leg.

3. Stand with your feet together, arms stretched out in front of you at shoulder level. Your palms should be facing down. Breathing in, rise up onto the balls of your feet. Concentrate on stretching and tightening your buttocks as you rise. Keeping your back straight, bend your knees and exhale while slowly descending to a squatting position. Repeat 10 times.

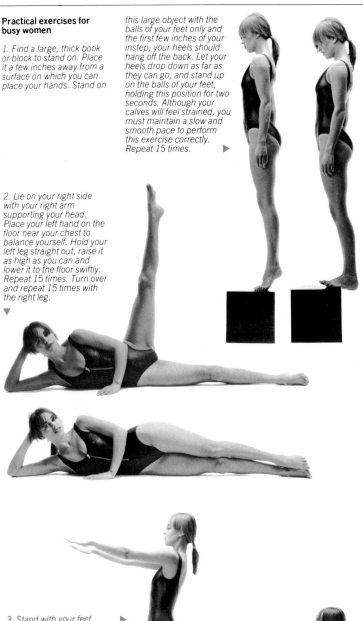

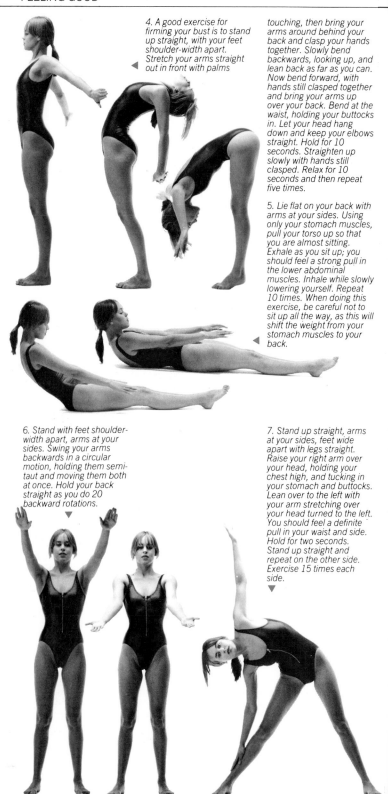

4. A good exercise for firming your bust is to stand up straight, with your feet shoulder-width apart. Stretch your arms straight out in front with palms touching, then bring your arms around behind your back and clasp your hands together. Slowly bend backwards, looking up, and lean back as far as you can. Now bend forward, with hands still clasped together and bring your arms up over your back. Bend at the waist, holding your buttocks in. Let your head hang down and keep your elbows straight. Hold for 10 seconds. Straighten up slowly with hands still clasped. Relax for 10 seconds and then repeat five times.

5. Lie flat on your back with arms at your sides. Using only your stomach muscles, pull your torso up so that you are almost sitting. Exhale as you sit up; you should feel a strong pull in the lower abdominal muscles. Inhale while slowly lowering yourself. Repeat 10 times. When doing this exercise, be careful not to sit up all the way, as this will shift the weight from your stomach muscles to your back.

6. Stand with feet shoulder-width apart, arms at your sides. Swing your arms backwards in a circular motion, holding them semi-taut and moving them both at once. Hold your back straight as you do 20 backward rotations.

7. Stand up straight, arms at your sides, feet wide apart with legs straight. Raise your right arm over your head, holding your chest high, and tucking in your stomach and buttocks. Lean over to the left with your arm stretching over your head turned to the left. You should feel a definite pull in your waist and side. Hold for two seconds. Stand up straight and repeat on the other side. Exercise 15 times each side.

**Flattening and toning your soft spots** Of over 600 muscles in the human body, the stomach muscles are often the most under-used. They require daily flattening and toning if you are serious about shaping a better body for yourself. When done correctly, the exercises will make you feel a slight burning sensation in your stomach. This tells you that the muscles are toning up, and that you are probably burning off some of the fatty tissue that surrounds them.

*1. Lie flat on your back with your arms spread wide on the floor. Slowly raise your legs straight up so that they are vertical, pointing your toes (looking at it from the side your body should form an 'L' shape.) After raising your legs, you must then lower them slowly all the way to the floor. Repeat 15 times. After two weeks, you should be able to do 20.*

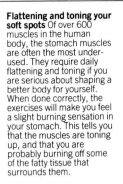

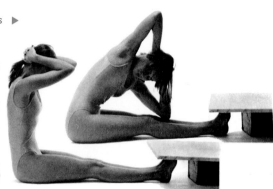

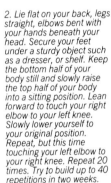

*2. Lie flat on your back, legs straight, elbows bent with your hands beneath your head. Secure your feet under a sturdy object such as a dresser, or shelf. Keep the bottom half of your body still and slowly raise the top half of your body into a sitting position. Lean forward to touch your right elbow to your left knee. Slowly lower yourself to your original position. Repeat, but this time touching your left elbow to your right knee. Repeat 20 times. Try to build up to 40 repetitions in two weeks.*

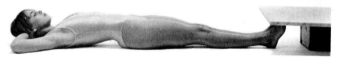

**Along with soft stomachs,** flabby thighs, hips and buttocks are also common figure problems. Toning these body areas is of major importance to the aspiring model, or any woman who wants to fit better into her jeans or bathing suit. The exercises below are excellent for slimming and strengthening. Again, try to build your stamina up so that you can increase the number of repetitions each day.

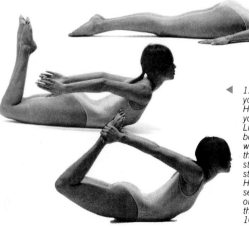

*1. Lie on your front with your head lifted off the floor. Holding your arms behind you, lift them to your sides. Lift your legs and upper body and bend them to-wards each other as far as they will go. Only your stomach and hips should still be touching the floor. Hold this position for three seconds and return to the original position. Rest for three seconds and repeat 10 times.*

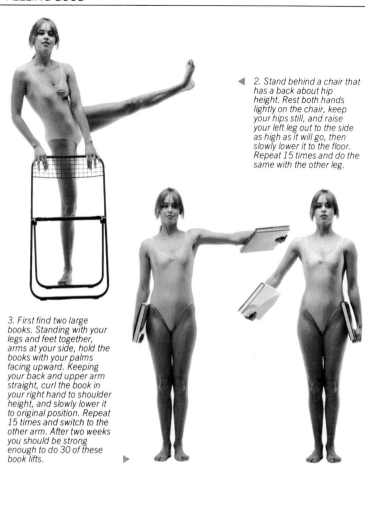

2. Stand behind a chair that has a back about hip height. Rest both hands lightly on the chair, keep your hips still, and raise your left leg out to the side as high as it will go, then slowly lower it to the floor. Repeat 15 times and do the same with the other leg.

3. First find two large books. Standing with your legs and feet together, arms at your side, hold the books with your palms facing upward. Keeping your back and upper arm straight, curl the book in your right hand to shoulder height, and slowly lower it to original position. Repeat 15 times and switch to the other arm. After two weeks you should be strong enough to do 30 of these book lifts.

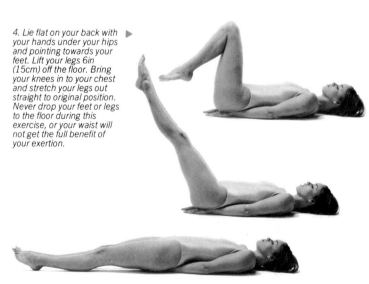

4. Lie flat on your back with your hands under your hips and pointing towards your feet. Lift your legs 6in (15cm) off the floor. Bring your knees in to your chest and stretch your legs out straight to original position. Never drop your feet or legs to the floor during this exercise, or your waist will not get the full benefit of your exertion.

# The sporting life

You may want to supplement your fitness routines with one or more sporting activity. Many models take aerobic dance classes to stay in shape because 'aerobic' or oxygen-using exercise, is one of the best ways to steadily develop physical and mental stamina. The opposite of aerobic exercise is anaerobic exertion, which includes such activities as lifting weights, playing golf, or walking. Aerobic exercise gets your lungs, heart and blood working faster, sending more oxygen and blood around the body to improve circulation and stamina. An hour of strenuous aerobic dancing can burn up to 600 calories; an hour of vigorous running can burn up to 900 calories. Other excellent aerobic sports include swimming, which burns up about 500 calories an hour, bicycling, which can burn up 660-700 calories an hour, and squash which burns up 600 calories in an hour of hard play. Roller skating is another aerobic sport. It can burn up nearly 500 calories an hour. Compare these workouts to anaerobic activities like golf, which burn up 220 calories an hour, or brisk walking, which only burns off 300 calories in an hour. Although you'll be using many different muscles during any given anaerobic activity, you will not increase your stamina with this kind of exercise because it does not involve the heart and lungs to such an extent.

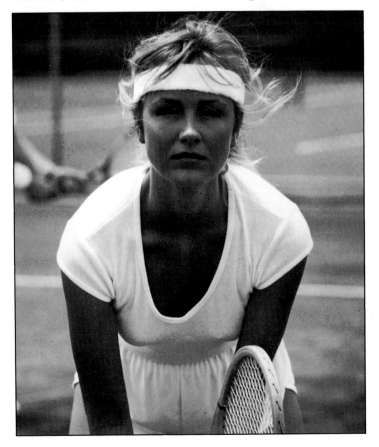

*Like squash, tennis is an excellent form of aerobic exercise.*

## How to relieve headaches

Headaches are a common affliction, triggered by stress, hunger, tension, a sudden drop in barometric pressure, lack of sleep and various other factors. One of the best and most natural ways to alleviate a headache is by breathing exercises. If you breathe deeply and rhythmically and then slowly exhale, you will bring more oxygen to your brain and your headache will disappear.

## The effect of hormones

It is well established that a woman experiences fluctuating hormone levels as a matter of course throughout each monthly menstrual cycle. Varying degrees of hormonal activity can alter mood, performance and appearance. Some of the more common symptoms of premenstrual hormone activity are sore, swollen breasts, irritability, depression, tension and general anxiety. Many women also experience a heavy, bloated feeling, lower backache and minor skin blemishes. Headaches, tearfulness and slight weight gain also number among the symptoms collectively known as 'premenstrual syndrome', or PMS. If you are afflicted with some (or many of) these symptoms during the 7-10 day interval before your period, there are measures that you can take to lessen their severity. Recent research into PMS indicates that frequent exercise (at least a half hour of activity four times a week or more) significantly reduces the amount of tension and anxiety that many women experience at the onset of their period. If your symptoms impair your ability to work and cause you severe discomfort, then you should see a gynecologist about the problem. Do not attempt to treat it yourself: it may be that your hormone levels need to be adjusted through specially prescribed hormone therapy.

## Saunas and massage

Saunas are a common feature of exercise clubs and gymnasiums, as their intense, dry heat improves blood circulation, relieves sore muscles, and cleanses the skin through profuse perspiration. A fifteen-minute sauna can also alleviate emotional tension and anxiety, leaving you mentally refreshed and calm. Saunas also help to exfoliate, or slough off, dead layers of skin, leaving it feeling

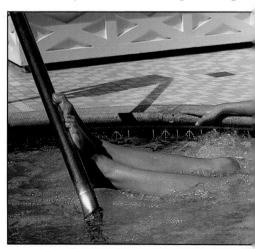

*Filled with water jets, the jacuzzi bath massages your body as you float. Its whirlpool-like action is excellent therapy for strained muscles and ligaments, sore feet and legs, arthritis and lower back troubles.*

softer and smoother. Because saunas can be a strain on the heart, do not enter one if you have any kind of heart condition. Also, do not enter a sauna room until you have completely cooled down from your workout and are breathing normally.

Swedish massage is the most commonly practiced form of massage in health and exercise clubs. The masseur, or masseuse, will massage parts of your naked body in careful order, starting with the legs and feet. Simultaneously stimulating and relaxing, massage strokes are always directed towards the heart. This is done to facilitate the flow of blood to the heart. Massage stimulates circulation and, by improving and nourishing the blood supply to the tissues, it quickens the healing process.

Another popular form of massage is the jacuzzi bath, which is a specially designed tub filled with water jets, which massage your body as you float. The whirlpool-like action of the jacuzzi is excellent therapy for strained muscles and ligaments, sore feet and legs, arthritis and lower back troubles.

## A good night's sleep

Sleep requirements vary from person to person, although it is generally agreed that most of us need a minimum of seven to eight hours a night. A sleepless night can impair your concentration, your vision and your motor coordination, besides affecting your mood and nerves adversely. John Hoffman, a nutritionist and biochemist who practices in New York, claims that it is not a good idea to stay up all night and then go to work. Regular sleep is crucial to a healthy lifestyle, he counsels, 'yet many people simply refuse to take this to heart. They think they're indestructible, but they're doing damage to themselves even if they don't realize it. Missing sleep always undermines the body and mind.'

For insomnia sufferers, John recommends a cup or two of strongly steeped peppermint tea. Health food stores often sell relaxing teas and natural sedatives. However, if you find yourself wide awake at 3 o'clock in the morning and you have no calming herbal teas in the cupboard, run a hot bath and soak in it for 10 minutes with the lights out and your eyes closed.

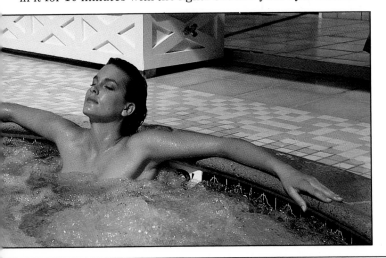

# HEALTHY EATING

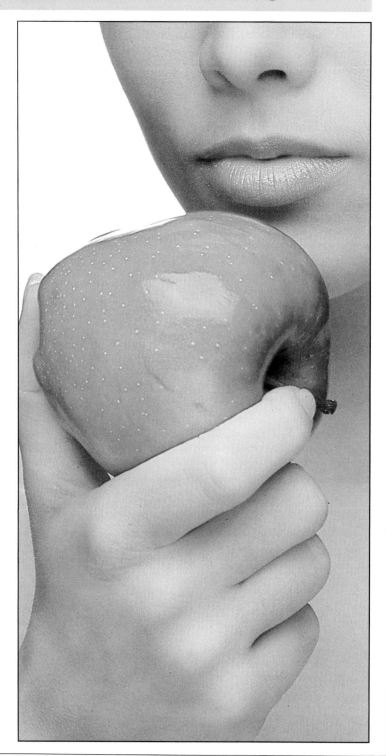

Whether you are an aspiring model or not, you need to develop intelligent eating habits. No one food contains all the nutrients, so a varied diet is essential. Contrary to popular opinion, modeling is a physically strenuous profession. Models are often expected to stand still for hours on end, hold their bodies in a variety of athletic poses, and walk gracefully down the catwalk in clothes that are sometimes very uncomfortable. This kind of work can be grueling if a model is improperly nourished or lacking in stamina. The following sections on diet offer advice from professional models on getting the most from your food.

The effect of food on the complexion is a hotly debated topic in doctor's offices and beauty magazines. Many people believe that fried foods, chocolate and cigarette smoking are some of the prime causes of acne pimples. Unfortunately, body chemistry is not as simple as this. Hormones are responsible for producing pimples and blackheads, and the only way that you can alter your hormone activity is by taking prescribed medication and this may only help temporarily. Some people find that certain foods make their skin look pale, spotty or pimply whenever they eat them. This could mean that they have a mild food allergy, and should avoid that particular food in the future. Some dermatologists recommend that processed and chemically preserved foods should be eliminated from the diet since artificially treated foods are unhealthy and have been known to cause allergic skin reactions in some people. In the final analysis, the best route to a rosy complexion is a simple one: a natural, well-balanced diet, coupled with daily exercise. Six to eight glasses of mineral water a day will also help to eliminate toxins from the body and keep your complexion clear.

You should eliminate the following foods from your diet because of their high fat content and calorie count: butter, fried foods, cake, candy, canned fruit in syrup, chocolate, biscuits, cream, dried fruit, honey, jam and jelly, mayonnaise, molasses, nuts, potato chips, puddings, salad dressing and refined sugar. Also cut down on the consumption of alcohol; it can cause puffiness, especially under the eyes. Processed foods (and these include canned goods, frozen foods and vegetables, breads, biscuits and cheese) are laden with salt. Recent studies have linked the use of salt to hypertension, high blood pressure and other illnesses.

You should eat as much bran and wheatgerm as you want. Wheatgerm is one of the few foods that contain vitamin E, all of the B vitamins except B12, along with potassium, magnesium, zinc and iron. It increases stamina, fights stress and fatigue and can be sprinkled into or onto everything you cook; the delicious nutty flavor goes well with eggs, vegetables, fruit salads, soups and meat dishes.

*The best route to a rosy complexion is via a natural, well-balanced diet (to include plenty of fresh fruit and up to eight glasses of mineral water a day).*

## Balancing your diet

Food can be divided into five major groups: cereals; dairy products; fats and oils; meat, fish and protein; fruits and vegetables. Although many nutritionists claim that you must eat foods from each of these groups to fulfil a minimum daily nutritional requirement, you should be aware that recent nutritional studies show a definite correlation between fat intake and rates of cancer of the breast and colon. It is wise, therefore, not only to cut your consumption of saturated fats (these are in all meat and whole-milk products), but to also reduce consumption of unsaturated fats, which are found in vegetable oils. It has also been proven that smoked, pickled and salt-cured foods increase the incidence of cancer in humans.

A balanced diet would include fresh fruit and vegetables; a low fat intake; a protein intake of 1¾oz (50g) per day; cereal such as bran and wheatgerm; lean fish or meats; and carbohydrates, which are found in sugar and starches. Another component of a balanced diet is water — you should drink at least four glasses a day. Mineral water is far healthier for you than tap water, which contains certain impurities.

## Vegetarian and vegan diets

There are two kinds of vegetarian: ovo-lacto vegetarian and vegan. The first group eats no animal flesh, but does eat animal products, such as cheese, milk, yogurt and eggs. Vegans eat only vegetables, fruits, grains and nuts, and no animal products. All vegetarians should supplement their diet with vitamins, such as desiccated liver, vitamin B12 or vitamin D and plan their meals carefully to ensure that the body's protein requirements are satisfied. Foods rich in protein include legumes (beans, peas and lentils) and grain (rice, wheat and corn). Vegans also need to eat plenty of foods that are high in iron, such as dark-green vegetables, watercress, whole grains and whole-grained breads; they must also keep up a high intake of calcium, which is found in all green vegetables and in sesame seeds. Finally, there is one food that is extremely high in protein and low in fat that vegetarians can combine with all vegetables; this is soybean curd, or tofu. It is excellent in soups or by itself with a little honey on top.

### HIGH-ENERGY, LOW-CALORIE DRINKS

**Cranberry Cooler**
*Cranberry juice, a splash of soda water and a leaf of crushed mint make a re-vitalizing drink. Besides giving you a quick lift, cranberry juice is a natural diuretic and thus cleanses your system.*

**Banana Malt**
*You'll need a blender for this one. Slice up a banana, add a glass of skimmed milk, a tablespoon of honey and a tea-spoon of wheatgerm. Blend until smooth and enjoy as a breakfast drink or as a snack.*

**Refresher**
*Mineral water with a citrus twist refreshes both body and mind without costing you any calories. Its prime health advantage is that it provides a natural 'lift' with none of the irritable side-effects of caffeine beverages. For more energy, cut down on your coffee or tea intake and drink mineral water throughout the day to effectively cleanse and replenish your system.*

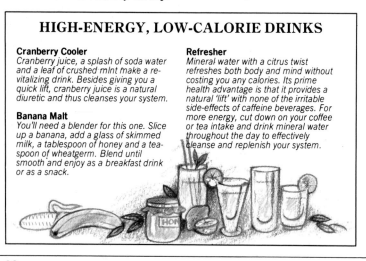

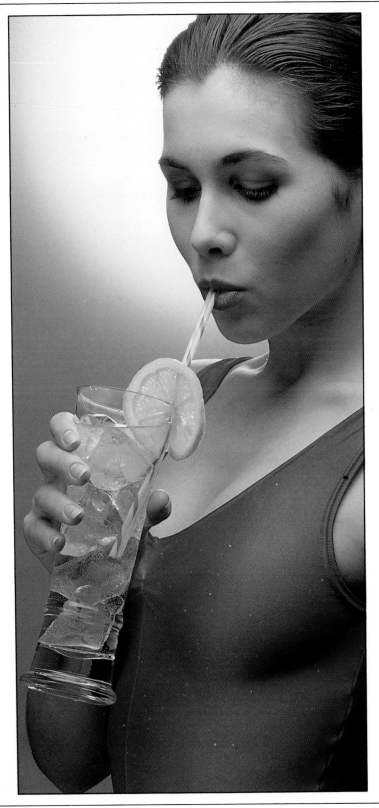

## A Model's Diet

By now you must realize that staying in shape and maintaining your looks — whether you are a heavily-booked model or an extremely busy person — demands that you strive to eat properly to keep fit. Beth Rubino, model and bodybuilder, has a broad knowledge of the body's biomechanics and nutrition. Here is her low calorie, low fat, high energy diet regime.

According to Beth, there is more to good nutrition than simply being selective about what you eat. 'You've got to listen to your body,' she explains. 'I'm a true advocate of eating only when you're hungry, for instance. I also think that you should reward yourself if you're craving a particular food, rather than constantly denying your body anything it's crying out for, whether it be sugar, pasta or whatever. My only hard and fast rules are: never eat large meals, never eat salt, processed foods or white sugar, and never, never eat before going to sleep at night. Your body cannot sleep and digest at the same time. The reason why I warn against large meals is because the body is not designed to digest large amounts of food at one time. Nu-

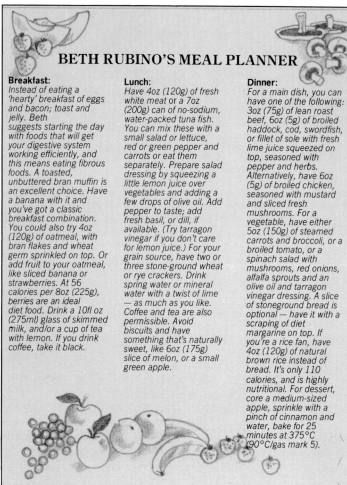

## BETH RUBINO'S MEAL PLANNER

**Breakfast:**
Instead of eating a 'hearty' breakfast of eggs and bacon; toast and jelly. Beth suggests starting the day with foods that will get your digestive system working efficiently, and this means eating fibrous foods. A toasted, unbuttered bran muffin is an excellent choice. Have a banana with it and you've got a classic breakfast combination. You could also try 4oz (120g) of oatmeal, with bran flakes and wheat germ sprinkled on top. Or add fruit to your oatmeal, like sliced banana or strawberries. At 56 calories per 8oz (225g), berries are an ideal diet food. Drink a 10fl oz (275ml) glass of skimmed milk, and/or a cup of tea with lemon. If you drink coffee, take it black.

**Lunch:**
Have 4oz (120g) of fresh white meat or a 7oz (200g) can of no-sodium, water-packed tuna fish. You can mix these with a small salad or lettuce, red or green pepper and carrots or eat them separately. Prepare salad dressing by squeezing a little lemon juice over vegetables and adding a few drops of olive oil. Add pepper to taste; add fresh basil, or dill, if available. (Try tarragon vinegar if you don't care for lemon juice.) For your grain source, have two or three stone-ground wheat or rye crackers. Drink spring water or mineral water with a twist of lime — as much as you like. Coffee and tea are also permissible. Avoid biscuits and have something that's naturally sweet, like 6oz (175g) slice of melon, or a small green apple.

**Dinner:**
For a main dish, you can have one of the following: 3oz (75g) of lean roast beef, 6oz (5g) of broiled haddock, cod, swordfish, or fillet of sole with fresh lime juice squeezed on top, seasoned with pepper and herbs. Alternatively, have 6oz (5g) of broiled chicken, seasoned with mustard and sliced fresh mushrooms. For a vegetable, have either 5oz (150g) of steamed carrots and broccoli, or a broiled tomato, or a spinach salad with mushrooms, red onions, alfalfa sprouts and an olive oil and tarragon vinegar dressing. A slice of stoneground bread is optional — have it with a scraping of diet margarine on top. If you're a rice fan, have 4oz (120g) of natural brown rice instead of bread. It's only 110 calories, and is highly nutritional. For dessert, core a medium-sized apple, sprinkle with a pinch of cinnamon and water, bake for 25 minutes at 375°C (90°C/gas mark 5).

tritionists are concluding more and more that you're better off eating five times a day — in small portions — than three huge meals. Salt is no good for you because it causes water retention and bloating, so, if you're a model like me, you simply shouldn't eat salt.'

When you are eating to control your weight, you may occasionally suffer from hunger pangs or feel dissatisfied after a meal. You can avoid these situations by filling up with mineral or spring water (six to eight glasses a day), and by eating plenty of raw vegetables. According to Beth, 'Vegetarians often have denser and thicker bones than people who follow meat-based diets. This is because green vegetables, especially the dark-green leafy ones, are loaded with calcium. The denser your bones are, the less chance there is that they'll break when you reach old age. It's something to think about now, while you still have a chance to build a strong body...Another thing you should be aware of is that sautéd and fried vegetables are robbed of their nutrients by the cooking process and, in addition to this, they're filled with empty calories. Boiled vegetables also lose a great deal of their vitamins in the process, so if you must cook your vegetables, stick to lightly steaming them for a few minutes. Otherwise, eat them raw in salads or as in-between meal snacks.

'If you can afford it, do try to visit a nutritionist so that you can determine what kind of vitamin supplements your body needs. I think proper eating habits should be one of everyone's major concerns, but obviously not everyone in our society is presented with the chance of learning how to live a healthier life...If you can afford to eat well and take vitamin supplements, then you should consider yourself fortunate.'

## Beth's raw vegetable snacks

You can eat as much as you want of the following vegetables, providing they are raw, or lightly steamed without sauces or butter: bean sprouts, artichokes, asparagus (it's a natural diuretic, meaning that it flushes fluids and toxins from your system), broccoli, brussels sprouts, cabbage, carrots, cauliflower, celery, green beans, all kinds of lettuce, mushrooms, green, red and white onions, red and green peppers, radishes, spinach, tōfu (also known as bean curd or soybean curd), tomatoes, turnips and watercress.

## How to stick to your diet when eating out

Beth has learned to resist the temptation of ordering the fattening dishes that appear on restaurant menus. 'Don't be prevented from asking for something broiled or poached to order,' she says. 'If you explain that you're on a limited diet, you'll never be refused. Another thing I always do is to inquire whether the restaurant's vegetables are fresh or frozen. I absolutely refuse to order them if they're frozen.' Desserts rich in calories, like cakes, pies, ice cream and puddings, are to be ignored. 'Have coffee or tea for dessert, and if you really crave something sweet, maybe you can arrange to have some fresh fruit.'

## Diet foods and slimming snacks

There are many dried breads and crackers on the market that are extremely low in calories (most of them have calorie information on the labels). You should eat these instead of regular bread, which is twice as fattening. Wild game is the leanest meat there is, and is a good source of protein for people who do not want to ingest the extra calories contained in beef or other fattier meats. Small portions of pasta are permissible — but don't combine pasta with a high carbohydrate side dish, such as potatoes. A few examples of other foods that are low in calories and good for dieting are: fresh fruit and vegetables, herbs and spices, popcorn (popped in an air popper only), natural plain yogurt, tuna fish packed in water and raw fish. You should also try to drink mineral water instead of diet sodas, some of which contain ingredients that have been linked to the development of bladder cancer in animals and humans. Diet sodas do however come in sodium-free flavors and, if you want to drink

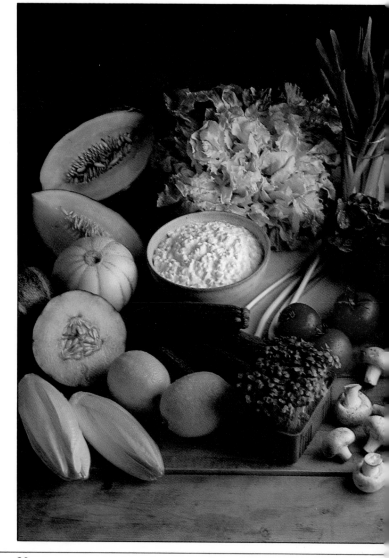

them, check the label before buying. Instead of white bread, eat whole-grained bread like stoneground wheat, rye and pumpernickel. These stimulate the colon to digest your food more efficiently.

No matter how well you plan your diet, there will be times when you will want a snack. Be prepared for food cravings by always keeping carrot, celery, and green pepper sticks sliced and ready for eating in between meals. Other sensible snacks include apples, cherries, strawberries, radishes, raw broccoli and cauliflower, grapefruits and oranges. Pour a tall glass of mineral water with a twist of lime for a zesty drink that will help curb your appetite. There is also a myriad of dietetic food products on the market, but these often contain chemicals and preservatives that are best avoided.

*A healthy diet can do more for your complexion than any cosmetics.*

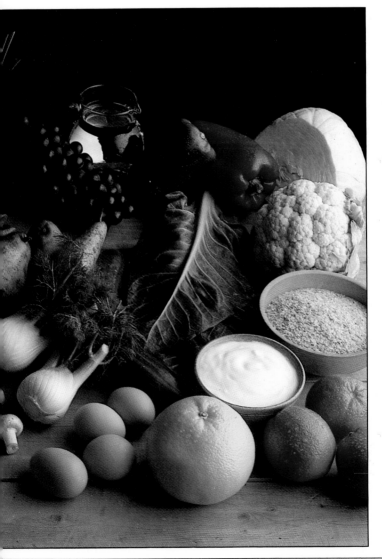

# 2
# LOOKING GOOD

*V*ery few people are blessed with a flawless complexion and perfectly proportioned features. Although heredity is the prime factor that determines your looks, all women can improve upon their natural assets with a little effort and some expert guidance. Elements of everyday life, such as cold weather, strong sunlight, pollution, smoking, drinking alcohol, central heating and air conditioning, have a detrimental effect on your skin, eyes, hair and teeth. Looking good means knowing how to overcome these factors, as well as being willing to devote some time to caring for your body.

# SKIN CARE

Besides being the largest organ of the body, your skin is one of the most sensitive registers of your physical health. Making the most of your complexion necessitates frequent exercise, sensible eating habits, and an appropriate skin-care routine. Although your skin type can never be altered, a well-organized, thorough skin-care program will make it look its best.

To discover your skin type, first remove all makeup from your face with a hypoallergenic soap. Hypoallergenic products do not contain sensitizers, such as lanolin or mineral oil and are therefore purer than other products. They are also scent-free and contain only the mildest ingredients so they are suitable for all skin types, and are especially good for sensitive skins. Next, rinse your face with tepid water. Do not use any astringent or moisturizer at this stage, but let your skin dry naturally. Now examine your face in natural light with a magnifying mirror — this will show the condition of your skin more accurately than a regular mirror. Look for areas of dryness, oily patches and any other indicators of skin type.

**Normal skin**
Ann Soorikian, New York beauty editor and author, claims that normal skin is quite rare. 'A normal skin is neither too oily, nor too dry. It's a well-balanced skin that is not affected by changes in climate, cosmetics or moods...Normal skin is not necessarily stronger than any other type, but it is more supple, smooth and evenly textured, with small pores.'

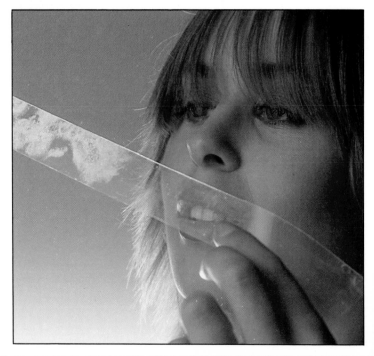

# Combination skin

Most of us have combination skin, with oily areas on the forehead, nose and chin. Dry areas tend to be around the eyes, and on the cheeks and throat. Black skins often have greater extremes of oiliness and dryness. If the contrast between dry and oily areas is severely pronounced on your face, you must be careful to employ different products on these patches. The dry areas should be washed with alcohol-free moisturizing cleansers, and moisturized regularly; the oily areas should be washed with light cleansers and alcohol-based astringents. If you have combination skin, use a mild, milky cleansing cream or lotion over the whole face. Rinse and towel dry. Any astringent that you use for oily spots should be diluted with water for the dryer parts of your face. Witch hazel is an inexpensive and effective astringent; so too are alcohol-free toners. Toners are less harsh astringents and are thus useful for more sensitive skin types. Apply toner with cotton cosmetic pads.

# Oily skin

If your face has an obvious shine to it, then your skin is oily. Other characteristics are a slightly sallow complexion and an uneven texture, due to open or overactive sebaceous glands. The shine on your face is caused by the overproduction of sebum, which is stimulated by the male hormone, androgen. Oily skin needs water to cleanse it and should be washed regularly with a soapless cleansing complexion bar or a granulated cleanser. After washing your face, be sure to rinse repeatedly with lukewarm water. Hot water will open your pores too much, allowing more dirt and particles to invade and irritate the sebaceous glands to produce more sebum. A final rinse with cold water will seal the pores. Next take a cotton ball or cotton cosmetic pad that is soaked in astringent and apply it all over your face, avoiding the eye area. Although vigorous cleansing is required to control oily skin, do not be too harsh. Scrubbing the face, or applying astringent too frequently can rob the skin of essential oil, causing flaking and producing blemishes. A facial brush or shaving brush is a good way to clean oily skin. You will probably not need a moisturizer, unless you live in a dry climate, but you should pay attention to sensitive areas, such as hands and elbows, during winter.

*To find out whether you have an oily, dry or combination skin, first cleanse your skin, remove excess oil and wait for half an hour. Then gently stick a five-inch strip of clear Sellotape across the bridge of your nose and gently peel it off. If it is covered with an even, slightly wet-looking sheen, your skin is oily. If it is covered with little white flaky particles, your skin is dry. If it has both flaky bits and a wet sheen, then you have combination skin.*

## Dry skin

If your skin is dry, it will look and feel dry and it may even peel or flake; cold weather can chap it in a matter of hours. Avoid all alcohol-based skin products and stick with rich milky, hypo-allergenic creams and lotions and gentle toners, such as rosewater. You must moisturize the face, throat and skin surrounding the eyes regularly. If you wear makeup, you may want to use moisturizing foundation over a moisture base; this is thicker than normal moisturizer and should be applied afterwards. Avoid products such as night creams and throat creams; they will clog the pores and prevent your skin from breathing.

## Sensitive skin

Blondes, redheads, and fair-skinned people are particularly likely to have sensitive skins, although all of us must guard against sunburn, allergic foods and cosmetics that can irritate. Generally speaking, sensitive skin does not tan well and tends to burn or freckle. It is also the type of skin that reacts to irritant foods, drinks or cosmetics by breaking out in spots, rashes and blemishes. Sensitive skin often blushes and pales more obviously than other skin types — it strongly reflects both moods and internal health. Women with sensitive skin should wear only hypo-allergenic (additive-free) make-up and should clean their faces with hypo-allergenic soaps, lotions and creams. Special care should also be taken when moisturizing, as sensitive skin is often quite dry.

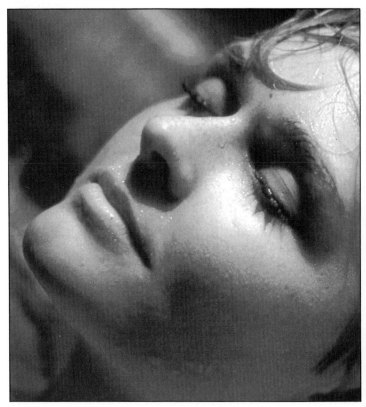

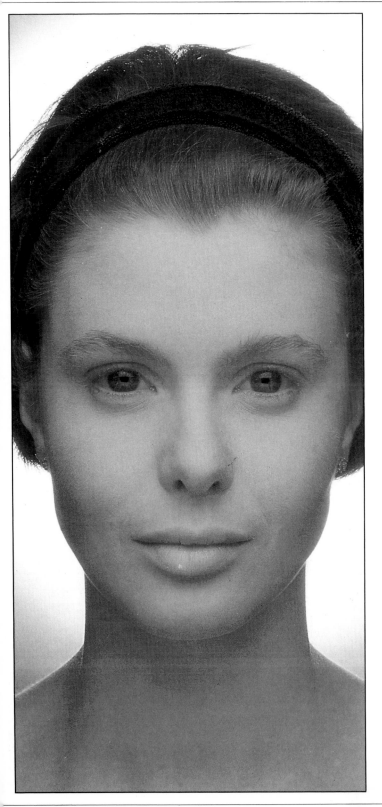

# FACIAL CLEANSING

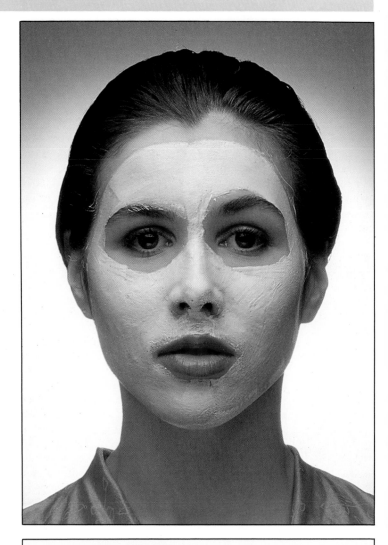

## HOME-MADE FACE MASK

**Directions for making**

*Wash and slice the cucumber. Grind it in a blender, skin and all. If you have no blender, grate cucumber in a bowl and catch all juice. Strain the juice through a clear nylon stocking or piece of muslin and set it aside. Throw away the pulp. You should now have the required amount of cucumber juice. Mix the egg whites and juice, beating with an electric beater until smooth. Then very slowly add the vodka, lemon juice, peppermint extract, and honey, beating constantly. This mixture makes about a cup of mixture. For a clingier, more tightening effect that helps cleanse oily skin, add 1½ to 2 egg whites to the recipe.*

**Directions for use**

*Apply the mask with your fingertips, avoiding the eye area. Dot the mask near your hairline and lie down for 10 minutes. For total relaxation and refreshment, place cotton wool or cotton cosmetic pads that have been moistened with witch hazel over your eyes while the mask is working. When the time is up, remove the pads and blot your eyelids dry with clean pads. Rinse off the mask with warm water and finally rinse with cold water to cleanse the pores. Towel dry. Let your skin breathe for half an hour and apply a light moisturizer if you have dry skin or slightly dry patches on your face.*

Although makeup can turn good looks into great looks, it is not positively beneficial to your skin. Michael Fletcher, a freelance make-up artist and hair stylist says: 'Your skin needs to breathe after wearing make-up; I tell all my clients to try to go for at least two days a week without wearing any make-up on their face. In order to maintain a healthy complexion your pores must be aired every now and then.'

You must thoroughly remove make-up with a good cleanser after every wearing. If you sleep with your make-up on, you risk clogging your pores and otherwise harming your complexion. It is also worth noting that sleeping with your eye make-up on can result in puffy eyes, uncomfortable eye irritations and even dangerous infections. Your skin will look its best if you remember that even the most skilfully applied make-up cannot mask a complexion that has not been cared for.

There are several products for cleansing and stimulating your face — liquid make-up removers, soap and water, cleansers and toners. However, all that is really required for an effective facial care program is a mild cleansing cream or liquid make-up remover, eye make-up remover, and an astringent or alcohol-free toner. Naturally, your individual skin type and the amount of make-up that you wear will dictate the kind of cleansing products that you use. Although cleansing with soap and water is sufficient for most skins, use a cold cream or liquid make-up remover first if you have dry or sensitive skin or are wearing make-up. In fact, women who regularly wear full face make-up may want to rely on cold cream and tissues as their primary cleansing method. 'You have to be as gentle as possible when cleansing,' says Beth Rubino, a print and television model. 'I have oily skin, but I use cold cream and tissues as a remover. I find that it's easier on my face than using a cleansing lotion and water.' Beth also uses a water-based eye make-up remover for lids and lashes. Experiment with both cold creams and cleansing lotion to find which product suits your skin best. If you have normal skin, you can clean your face with whatever product you prefer: cold cream, liquid cleanser or a light, milky cleansing cream.

When cleansing a face that has not been made-up, there are different options for different skin types. For instance, if you have dry or sensitive skin, you may want to use a moisturizing, hypo-allergenic soap and water or, if your skin is ultra-delicate, a creamy liquid cleanser or cleansing cream may be more ap-

*Make a weekly facial scrub or mask treatment part of your beauty routine. Whether your skin is oily, dry, combination or sensitive, masks or scrubs will revitalize your skin by improving surface circulation, removing dead skin cells and cleansing the pores.*

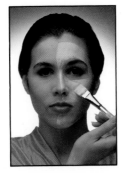
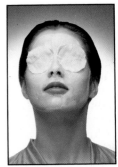

propriate. For normal skins you can use anything from a mild soap to liquid cleanser, following up with an alcohol-free toner. If you have oily skin, you could try a specially formulated soap that will help to dry out your skin, or a facial mask or scrub. After your cleansing routine, give your face a final touch of refreshment with a mineral water spray mist. These are available from drug stores; they make the skin tingle and feel smoother in seconds. Many women also use mineral water spray after making up. A few quick mists will add extra moisture and fix your eyeshadow and foundation.

## Deep cleansing

Facial masks and scrubs help in the cleansing, exfoliation and stimulation of specific skin types. Exfoliating scrubs and masks clean away the surface layer of dead cells that can clog the pores or give the skin a gray cast. Dead skin most often accumulates on the face, elbows, knees and feet, and these areas can be softened by regular use of a gritty scrub. You can make your own facial scrub with natural ingredients, such as oatmeal, lemon juice and herbs.

For intensive pore cleansing, consult a professionally licensed skin-care salon. Be sure to inquire about what methods they use for facial treatment before making an appointment. Steam, lotions, creams or hand massage are the safest and most effective methods of cleansing used in a professional facial.

## Moisturizers

After using toner and astringent to remove all traces of cleanser, the next step in your skin-care routine is moisturizing. Moisturizers act on the surface layers of the skin to protect them from moisture loss. They work in conjunction with the body's natural oil — sebum — to lubricate the skin and protect it from the elements. All moisturizers are essentially water and oil mixtures; the greater the ratio of oil in the product, the thicker the moisturizer will be. Remember that the heavier the cream, the harder it is for the skin to absorb. Thus, if you're looking for light moisturizers, stick to water-based products. If you have a normal or combination skin, a light, water-based moisturizer should be all you need underneath your make-up and on dry areas of your body. If you have dry skin, you will want some kind of oil-based cream or lotion. If you have sensitive skin, be sure to use a hypo-allergenic moisturizer that does not irritate.

Although many advertisements for moisturizers claim that these products can rejuvenate and regenerate skin cells, this is not the case. The only way you can nourish your skin is by eating healthy food, drinking several glasses of water a day, and getting plenty of vitamins. Furthermore, moisturizers or cosmetic products labeled 'biologically active' or 'bio-energetic' are in no way superior to any other product. Magazine beauty editor Anne Soorikian explains, 'It is a current trend in the cosmetics industry to introduce "high-tech" cosmetics. Although the use of the "bio-" prefix implies scientific properties and sounds very modern, all "bio-" really means is that the product is designed for use on and by a living being!'

# COMMON SKIN PROBLEMS

Many of us at one time or another experience minor skin problems such as acne, allergic rashes and blemishes. These occasional flare-ups can be treated with off the shelf preparations, but if they frequently recur or become more pronounced with time, you should see a dermatologist. The chart above gives guidelines for treating and masking some of the more common skin problems.

### Acne

*If you have periodic outbreaks of acne, such as before your menstrual period or during times of stress, the best thing you can do to keep blemishes and oiliness under control is to wash the skin twice daily with a soap or cleanser that is formulated for oily skin. Wipe only the oily areas with a medium-strength astringent. Never try to squeeze your blemishes, as this will spread the infection and cause more blemishes to erupt. If your pores are large and you want to discourage blackheads and whiteheads, use a medium-strength astringent four times a day. Be careful not to use one that is too strong, as it may cause your pores to produce more oil. There are several medicated acne cover-up cakes and creams on the market that are tinted to match different skin tones. Although these will not make your blemishes invisible, they will make them less obvious as well as help to dry them out.*

### Inflamed skin

*These conditions are triggered by a variety of factors, including allergies, overexposure to the sun, and emotional upset. Although only time will heal them, you can soothe and cover them up for the duration. If any of these conditions are accompanied by itching, however, you must see a doctor as soon as possible for diagnosis. Irritating rashes can be alleviated by holding a hot compress against the affected area for a half hour or more. If the skin is not unduly tender, you can try a technique advised by makeup artist Patrick Dennis. Blend in some liquid foundation, allow it to dry, and use a loose, translucent powder to cover. Apply the powder with a wide makeup brush, shaking off any excess before applying it to the skin.*

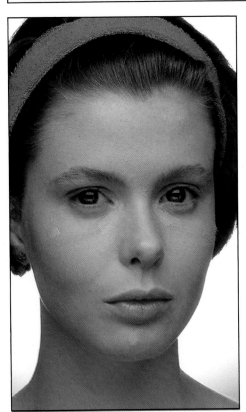

*There are several medicated acne cover-up cakes and creams on the market that are tinted to match different skin tones. As well as making blemishes less noticeable, they also help to dry them out.*

# MAKEUP

Now that you've mastered the skin-care basics and know how to treat your complexion, you may want to study the following makeup techniques. A section on body makeup is also included.

If your complexion is free of inconsistencies, perhaps you don't need any foundation or concealing cream. A simple dusting of blusher may be all the color your face requires to look its best. However, though women with oily skin should also use compressed powder to avoid a shine, if you want your face to have the matt finish of a professional model's, then you should practise using foundation or concealers for shadows under the eyes and other imperfections. If you have oily or combination skin, use water-based moisturizers, foundations and concealers. Women with dry skin should use oil-based foundations. In the summer, tanning creams and bronzing gels can also be quite useful for evening out your skin tone in areas that are peeling. They work by temporarily dyeing the skin. Some of these tanning products have been known to turn the skin an unsightly orange or rust shade so always test them on a small patch of skin before applying them all over. They are not recommended for use on sensitive skin, but if you can find one that is hypoallergenic (additive-free),  give it a try.

## Concealers

Concealer helps to disguise flaws, such as shadows or bags under the eyes, and can subtly brighten your face, if used on particular spots. Concealer is available in cover sticks, creams and cakes. The cover stick is the most popular with models because

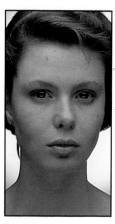

**Concealer**
*Concealer comes in light and tan tones. If you have dark skin, use tan; for medium or fair skin, choose light. Use the concealer sparingly — you do not want it to look too conspicuous.*

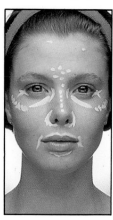

*Dot under eyes, in the middle of your forehead and just above the upper lip. Next put a dot down the centre of your nose and chin.*

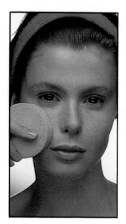

*Blend the concealer in with swift strokes to cover the skin. You can also blend some on the brow bone and underneath the eyebrows. This will make a good base for your makeup.*

it is easy to apply. If you have dry skin, however, you will probably prefer to use the cream.

Pimples or spots can easily be concealed. What you need in addition to your everyday liquid foundation and powder is solid foundation base in a slightly darker shade. Invest in a fine-tipped make-up brush for application. First apply foundation, then cover stick and powder. Paint the foundation base on to the pimple and blend into the rest of the foundation. Powder to set, and touch up as needed throughout the day.

Wrinkles, crow's feet and frown lines can be significantly softened through a three-step process. You must first select a stick of solid base in a pale tone. For instance, if you have a medium skin tone, try a fair or light-toned stick of base. Don't choose anything that will contrast markedly with your liquid foundation. You'll also need an eyeliner brush and cotton cosmetic pads. Apply your foundation and let it set for five minutes; now rub the eyeliner brush over the base, taking up a small amount of color. Paint a thin line inside the crease formed by the wrinkle and make sure the color is blended evenly. Set the powder, folding the cotton pad to ensure that the wrinkle gets completely powdered. For larger wrinkles or frown lines, apply the stick of base directly on to the skin and blend with fingertips, then set with powder.

## Foundation

Foundation comes in different forms — cream, cake, gel and stick — but liquid foundation is the easiest to apply. When selecting a foundation, look for one that is as close to your own skin tone as possible; you don't want to alter the color of your skin with foundation, you simply want to define it and make it look even. Remember when you test colors, try them on your face, not on your hands or forearms.

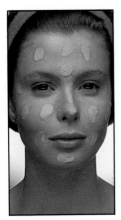
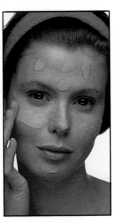
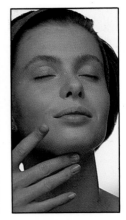

**Foundation**
*About five minutes before applying foundation, put a thin coating of moisturizer on your face. This will help to spread the colour evenly. Use a tiny, slightly damp sponge or fingertips to apply foundation.*

*Dot circles on eyelids, under eyes and on forehead. Also dot the centre of your nose, cheeks and under your chin.*
*Blend the liquid into your skin with a quick, light touch. Do not rub it in as this can clog the pores.*

*Blend the foundation onto your neck with long strokes that stop at the collar bone. Finally, take a tissue and cover your face lightly; the tissue will absorb any excess foundation. Lean your head forward and shake the tissue off.*

## Powder

Use translucent powder that is tinted to match your skin tone and foundation and apply it with a large cotton cosmetic pad or powder puff. Dip the pad gently into the powder and press very softly on to your face, making sure that the jawline, under-eye area and forehead are well covered. Use a makeup brush to dust off any excess. You have now set your foundation and achieved a model-perfect, matt texture.

If applying makeup for night wear, try dusting pearlized or metallic highlighting powder over your cheeks and forehead; bear in mind that a minimal amount is all that is needed for a special effect. Silver looks especially good on pale skins, while gold flecks on the eyes and earlobes create a high-voltage, glamorous look that dramatizes your eyes and ears. Black skins look dazzling with all shades of metallic glints. Experiment to find the right one for your coloring — you may discover some that go perfectly with day makeup, too.

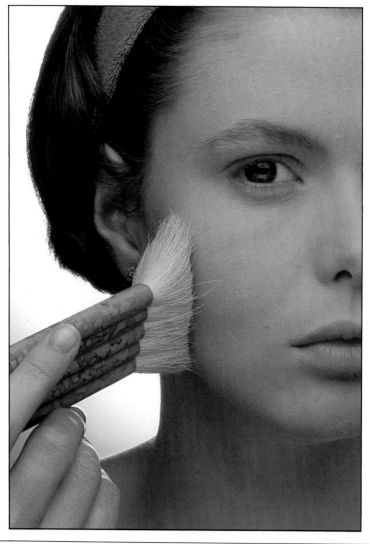

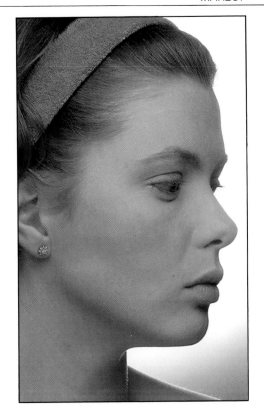

*Before applying contour makeup, it is important to assess your bone structure and the shape of your face. As a general principle, pale contours lighter than your skin tone emphasize bone structure, while darker colours make over-prominent features recede. Contour comes in the form of powders, gels, sticks and pencils. The powders are easiest to apply (see left) but you will need various sizes of makeup brush for different parts of your face.*

## Contour and makeup

The underlying principle of contour makeup is that pale colors lighter than your skin tone emphasize bone structure, while darker colors make over-prominent features recede. Applying contour color is a simple, easy-to-learn skill. Most professional models rely on contouring techniques to subdue minor facial imbalances, but if you simply want to look your best, then mastering appropriate contour skils is a worthy investment of time and energy.

Contour comes in compressed and loose powders, gels, sticks, and pencils. Like eyeshadows, the powders are easiest to apply and control in intensity. You will therefore need various sizes of makeup brush for different parts of your face. To clean the brushes after application, stroke them with a tissue, separating the hairs and shaking out any excess powder.

Your bone structure and the overall shape of your face will determine which contour makeup techniques are right for you. Begin then, by assessing the shape of your face. Take a long, objective look at your features and how they appear in relation to each other. If your face is wider than it is long, then you have a round or wide face. A face that is one and three-quarters longer than it is wide is considered long. If the width from one side of the jaw to the other is markedly less than the widest part of the face, and if the chin is narrow or pointed, then you have a heart-shaped face. If the proportions are the same but the jaw is blunt or somewhat square, then your face is square-shaped.

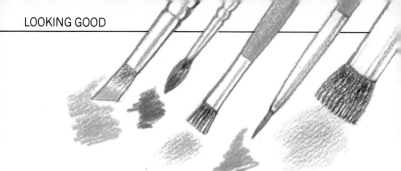

## Giving a large forehead better proportions

*Apart from styling your hair differently, there is no sure way to hide a large forehead, but it can be minimized and softened by shading with a rosy tone. Start at the temples, where the forehead gives way to the hairline. Blend well and apply more shading if necessary.*

## Changing the shape of your nose

*To narrow the bridge of the nose, draw a fine line with shader down the side of the nose from your eyebrow, stopping when you reach the level of the outer corner of your eye. Blend the shader carefully. To make your nose look slender, draw a fine line of shader down the side, beginning at the outer corner of the eye and stopping at the bottom of the nose just above the nostril. Again, blend carefully so that no tell-tale marks remain. If your nose looks too flat and you'd like to minimize this, brush a light brown blusher down either side and around the nostrils. Blend a thin line of highlighter down the front of your nose. To make large nostrils look smaller, apply shader in a thin line with an eyeliner brush in a crescent-moon shape around the crease at the side of each nostril. The contour should be widest and darkest at the nostril. Be sure to fade the line out at the edges.*

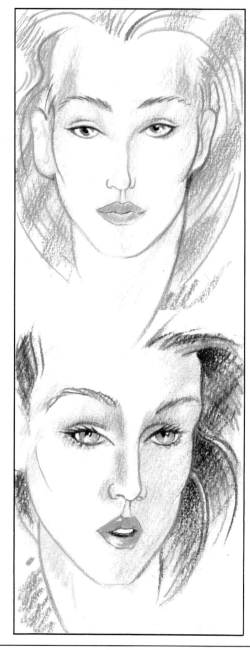

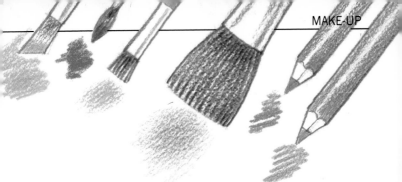

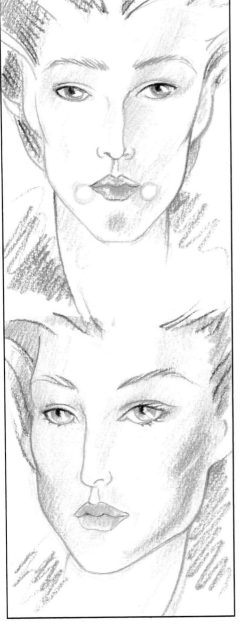

**Changing the shape of your chin**
To highlight a firm chin or re-define a receding one, brush cream-toned highlighter on the front of the chin and blend it in. To soften a pointed chin, apply highlighter under the outer corners of the mouth in the indentations at each side of your chin. Do not blend yet. Next, apply a quarter-sized dot of shader to the front of your chin and blend all three spots of color, starting with the shader.

**Narrowing a full face**
Apply shader on the fullest part of your cheeks, between the cheek and jawbones. Start the shader below the center of the eye and angle it upwards, towards the center of your ear. Blend well. Now brush on highlighter in a diagonal line above the cheekbones from the outer corner of the eye to the hairline. Widen the diagonal area as you work out towards the hairline and top of the ear. Blend the edges.

# EYE CARE

Before you begin experimenting with various eye makeup colors and techniques, look into a magnifying mirror to determine the shape of your eyes and eyebrows. Are your eyes small and deep-set, round or almond-shaped? Do they protrude slightly or droop? Are they close-set or wide-set? If you are Black or Oriental, your eyes are probably a striking shape that calls for a specific color combination and makeup technique.

Now examine your eyebrows. The perfect eyebrow should be nearly the same width all the way across. It should taper at the outer corner and fall into a natural line. In general, fine-boned features on a small face look best with a subtle brow, while strong features are balanced by thicker eyebrows. It is advisable not to change the natural shape of your eyebrows because the ideal brow is usually proportionate to the width and fullness of your facial features. Your eyebrows should also mirror the curve of your lash line.

## Reshaping eyebrows

If you think you need to define the shape of your eyebrows, first rid the eye area of oil or grime with an astringent. Next assemble the following: angle-tipped tweezers, an eyebrow brush, cotton cosmetic pads, witch hazel and alcohol. Before you tweeze, dip the tweezer tips into the alcohol — this will sterilize them and protect your skin from infection. Brush your eyebrows upwards and outwards with firm strokes. Always tweeze under the eyebrow, and place the tips as close to the base of the hair as possible. You want to pluck the entire hair shaft and root, otherwise you will be left with stubbly root hairs.

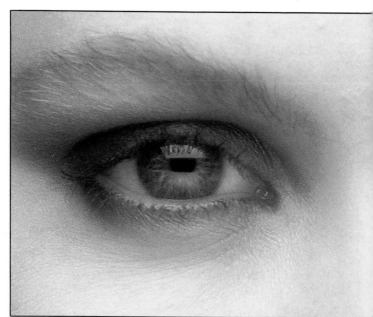

Check this area daily in your magnifying mirror for new growth.

While tweezing, hold the skin taut above the brow with your free hand. If your skin is sensitive, tweeze at night so any redness will have disappeared by morning. Remember that if you tweeze excessively, your eyebrows may never grow back again. Never tweeze above the brow, you want to shape your brows into a clean line, not prune them. After you've finished tweezing, wipe the area clean with pads soaked in witch hazel to clean and close the pores.

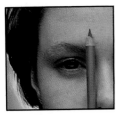
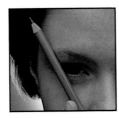
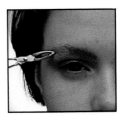

*To measure your eyebrows, hold a pencil vertically along the line of your nose. If your brow line overlaps onto the bridge of your nose, pluck the excess hair. If the line falls short, pencil it in.*
*To find out where the brow line should taper away, hold the pencil diagonally from the base of your nose across the outer corner of your eye.*

*The brow should finish in the same place as the tip of the pencil. If it falls short, pencil it in; if it overlaps, pluck it.*

*When plucking your eyebrows, carefully pluck both hair-shaft and root.*

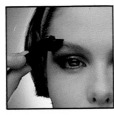
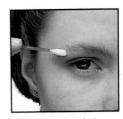

*Brush your eyebrows up-wards and outwards with firm strokes.*

*Rid the eye area of oil or grime with a cotton cosmetic pad.*

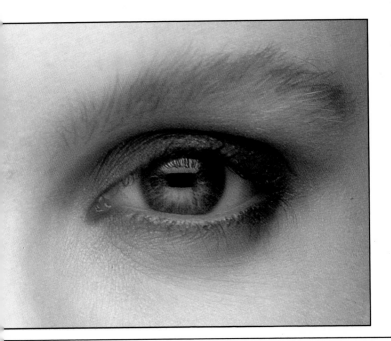

# Eye color: contouring and highlighting

Applying eye color is a simple way of contouring and highlighting your eyes. There are a few fundamental rules to follow when applying eye color. Use more than one eye shadow, for instance, if you want to have well-defined eyes with shape and depth. Line the inside lower rims of the eyes with kohl eyeline pencil to markedly brighten the whites of the eyes and emphasize them. Before beginning your eye makeup, always apply a concealing cream as needed around the eye area. Use your fingertips for blending it in. Next, set the eye area with a thin dusting of translucent powder. Remove excess by buffing with a cotton pad or small make-up brush. Because different eye shapes require specialized contouring techniques, here is a strategy for each specific eye shape.

### Small eyes

*If your iris (the colored part of your eye) is proportionally smaller than the white of your eye, then you have what are considered small eyes. To make them more prominent, brush on a light-colored, powdered eyeshadow with an angle-tipped brush just above your lashes. Apply a darker shadow near the crease. Do not color near the inner corner of your eye, for this will make your eyes look smaller. When applying shadow at the sides, use your brush to blend the powdered shades into one another. A light-gray eye pencil should be used under the eye to create a more open and wide-eyed look.*

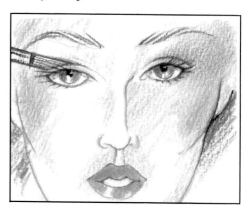

### Wide-set eyes

*With a small blusher brush, apply contour powder that is slightly darker than your skin tone, between the eyes and the bridge of your nose. Brush and blend the powder down the side of your nose. Practice this technique with your magnifying mirror until you perfect it. Next, brush a neutral-toned highlighter under the outside edge of the brow. Shade the crease line, emphasizing the inside corner of the eye. Finish by brushing a light matt shadow on the outer corner of the eye.*

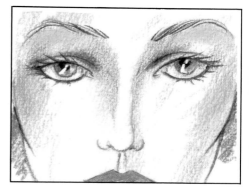

### Almond eyes

*Brush a light-coloured shadow on to your brow bone. Blend in a color that is a few shades darker on your eyelid. Line the lower inside rim of the eye with black or brown kohl pencil, extending the line out to the corner of your eye. If you have blue eyes, use a blue pencil.*

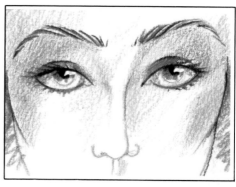

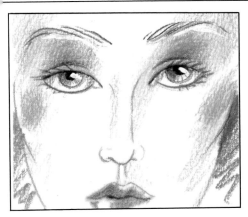

### Deep-set eyes
*To make deep-set eyes more prominent, brush a pale pink or beige shadow over the eyelid and fade it out above the hollow of the crease. Then apply a medium-toned eyeshadow starting at the brow bone and blending it up into the brow. Darken the eye area directly over the natural crease with a smoky-colored shadow that blends well with your other choices. Line the inside lower rim of the eye with black or brown pencil.*

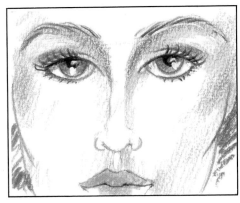

### Drooping eyes
*Brush a medium-toned shadow, starting at the inside corner of the eye, in an upward and outward stroke, stopping just short of the brow line. Do not brush any color on the outer edge of the lid where the eye begins to droop. Instead, create a crease line that is slightly higher than your own by shading it with taupe or medium-brown eyeshadow. Curling the lashes will make your eyes look less droopy, as will a few coats of mascara.*

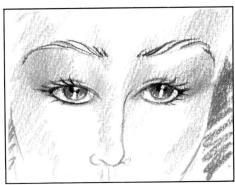

### Close-set eyes
*Brush a pale highlighter on the inside corner of your eyes — a white shadow would be fine for this — and blend it carefully into the side of the nose. This technique will make your eyes appear farther apart. Next, brush a dark-toned shadow on to the outside third of your brow bone, shaping upward and outwards. The final effect should look as if the dark-toned shadow is growing out of the corner of your eye, shading up across the brow bone and stopping at the outer edge of your eyebrow. If you want maximum definition, line the lower inside rim of your eyes with kohl pencil in black, or any other color that coordinates well with your eyeshadow.*

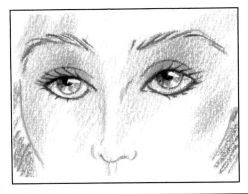

### Protruding eyes
*Shade the entire lid with a medium to deep-colored eyeshadow. Never use frosted shades or highlighters, as they will emphasize your prominent brow bones and protruding eye sockets. Blend shadow up on to the brow bone. Apply eyeliner pencil on the lower inside eye rims. Curling the eyelashes can help to de-emphasize protruding eyes; if you wear mascara, coat only the lashes in the centre of the lid.*

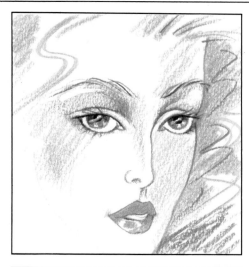

### Round eyes

*Choose a deep-hued shadow in any color. Apply shadow, starting at the inside corner of the eye. Blend the color in an upward angle towards the outer edge of the brow. Intensify the color in the corner of the eye and lessen it as you work up towards the brow. Apply a lighter-toned shadow or pencil under the lower lid, and extend the color up and out to blend with the color below. Dust a tiny amount of pale highlighter near the brow line.*

### Oriental eyes

*Brush a pale matt eye-shadow over the entire lid area. Pale pink would work well, as this happens to be a traditional eye color for Japanese and Chinese women. Next apply a medium-toned eyeshadow on the inner corner of the eye; intensifying the color closest to the bridge of the nose. Continue blending towards the center of your eye until the shadow fades out, then brush a darker shade of shadow on the outer corner of the eye. You want to keep the color most intense near the lid. Blend from the outer corner of your lid in an arc towards the outer edge of the eyebrow. Also blend subtly towards the nose to merge all the colors and define your eyes with this field of color.*

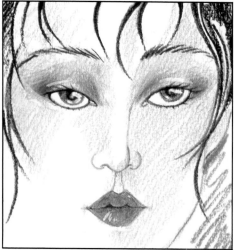

*Apply kohl eyeliner to the lower inside rims of the eyes. The finer the point of the eyeliner, the more depth it will give to your eyes. Apply eyeliner in a thin line because a slash of color will make your eyes seem heavy and slitted. Finally, smudge the area below the outside of the lower lashes with a kohl pencil in a subtle tone such as beige, grey or rose.*

### Eye makeup for Black women

*Apply a deep-toned shadow on the outer half of the eyelid. Brush a bright shadow on to the center of the lid and color all the way up under the brow. Line the inside lower rims of the eyes with blue kohl pencil. This will emphasize your eyes in a way that no other color can. Finish with two or more coats of mascara. Violet and blue look especially colorful on dark-skinned women. Experiment with highlighters under the brow for a different effect.*

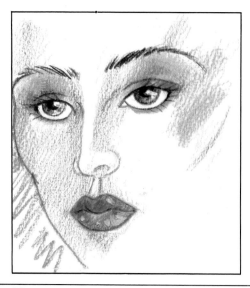

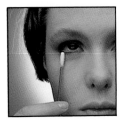

Apply eye-drops to soothe sore or bloodshot eyes.

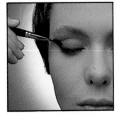

Define the eye area with a thin dusting of translucent powder.

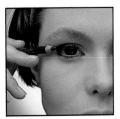

Draw a pencil line on inside of lower lid above the lash line.

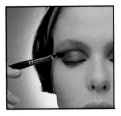

Apply a pale shade over the top lid with a sponge applicator.

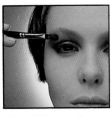

Highlight the brow line with a soft ivory shade.

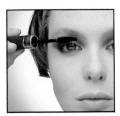

Apply mascara to the upper lashes, use zigzag movements for lower lashes.

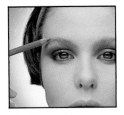

Carefully pencil in your eyebrow shape with light strokes.

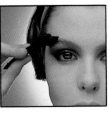

Brush eyebrows upwards into a gentle arch with a small brush.

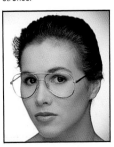

Spectacles are IN! If you wear them, remember to adapt your eye make-up so that it blends in with your frames — especially if they are brightly colored.

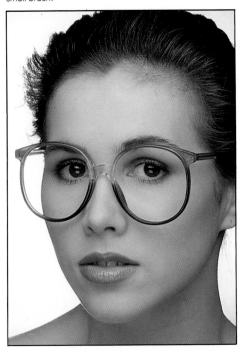

# EYESHADOW TO SUIT YOUR EYES

**Dark eyes**
*Try mauve, rose and silvery grey, canary yellow, beige and gold; ivory, navy blue and turquoise.*

**Hazel eyes**
*Pale brown, copper highlighter, rust brown; pale pink, lilac, deep purple; brown, silvery grey and khaki.*

**Green eyes**
*Gold highlighter, pale orange, red-gold; bone, bronze, khaki; and pale grey, electric blue and yellowy gold.*

**Brown eyes**
*Grey-blue, lilac, grape purple; salmon pink, pink-gold and deep rose; pale gold, brick red and medium brown.*

**Blue eyes**
*Pink-lilac, mauve highlighter, plum; white, greyish purple, dark grey; and white, jade and smoky blue.*

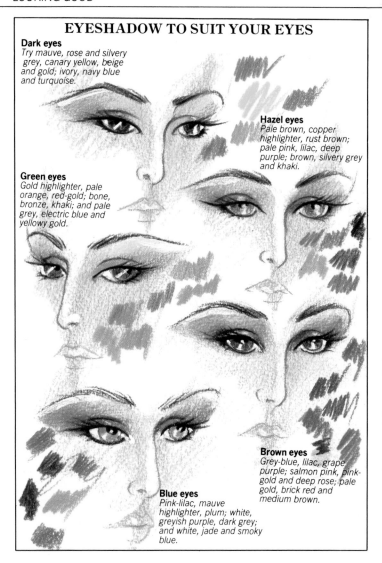

## Eyelashes

An aspect of eye care often overlooked involves the eyelashes. The average eyelash lives as long as four months. In its brief life span, it helps to protect your eyes by taking abuse from water, sun, make-up and pollution. To keep lashes lustrous and healthy, try dabbing on a drop of mineral oil before bedtime. The oil will safely soak and condition the hairs overnight and, in the morning, use a cotton cosmetic pad for removing all traces.

The simplest way to emphasize eyelashes is by curling them. An eyelash curler is quicker to use than mascara, and involves no cosmetics. Never apply mascara before curling or you risk painful damage to your lashes. To curl the lashes, take the curved wand and place it close to the base of the upper lash line. The upper lashes should come through the gap. Squeeze gently for six seconds. Thick lashes often need repeat squeezes. Do not curl the lower lashes.

*Successful make-up involves enhancing good features and disguising flaws while retaining a 'natural' look. A good foundation will protect your skin, disguise any uneven coloring and provide a base for powder. Eyes should be made to look larger and more radiant, lips fuller and softer.*

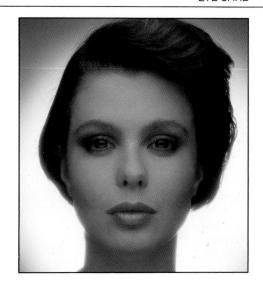

## A final word about eye care

Although eye color comes in many different forms, the powder eyeshadow, whether compressed or loose, is recommended by make-up artists and models because it is easiest to apply and control. It also lasts longer than creams, gels or crayons, which have a tendency to crease and fade quickly on normal to oily skins. Powdered eyeshadow tends to cake on older women, so they should use liquid eyeshadow. This comes in bottles and does not accentuate wrinkles as powder and cream eye-shadow sometimes do.

There are several products that you can use to remove eye makeup. The least irritating is an alcohol-free eye makeup remover lotion. There are also pre-soaked cotton pads on the market. Both the lotion and the pads are available in hypo-allergenic preparations. Another common eye makeup remover is baby oil; it is inexpensive and does not irritate the skin. Use it with cotton cosmetic pads and cotton swabs.

To remove eyeshadow, apply a thin veneer of remover to browbone and eyelids. Let it sink in for 30 seconds — this will help to dissolve the shadow. Wipe off with cotton wool or cotton cosmetic pads until they wipe clean. Use a cotton swab around the corners of the eye and place a small piece of tissue underneath your lashes. Wipe both upper and lower lashes with a cotton pad or cotton wool that is moist with remover. Use pads until they wipe clean. Wipe away any lingering particles of eye makeup or mascara with a cotton swab. Next, use a toner to cleanse your eye area and rinse with cold water to close pores. If you wear contact lenses, you must make special allowances for them when applying eyeshadow, mascara, and eye pencil. Products that you should avoid include waterproof mascaras, mascaras formulated with fibers, and loose eyeshadow powders. These can all flake off into the eye, causing discomfort or infection. Always select water-soluble mascara that has been hypoallergenically tested for irritants. Apply your eye makeup with a soft brush or cotton swab.

# LIP CARE

Even the most expertly applied makeup in the world cannot hide dry, chapped lips. You should care for your lips by moisturizing them regularly with petroleum jelly, clear lip gloss, or medicated lip balm. If you have a moisturizing lipstick, then that may be all you need. To make your lips look their best, you also want to take proper care of the rest of your mouth — namely, your teeth and gums. Brush your teeth after every meal, use dental floss, and visit your dentist for regular check-ups and teeth cleanings (see page 77 for dental care).

Because your mouth and lips are extremely prominent and expressive, you should do everything in your power to keep the muscles surrounding them relaxed. Tensing and pursing them will inevitably result in wrinkles and fine lines forming around your mouth. Here is a quick trick for relaxing your mouth and lips: with mouth closed, slowly puff up your cheeks with air. Then allow your lips to part so as to exhale a tiny, slow stream of air. As your mouth gradually deflates, your muscles will settle into their natural position.

Just as your face should be moisturized before you apply make-up, your lips also need a thin coating of moisturizer before applying lip color. The lips have no lubricating oil glands, and are often the driest parts of the body, especially if you are a smoker. Try to apply a lip salve every night before going to sleep. To remove lipstick, squirt some baby oil onto a paper tissue and wipe your lips.

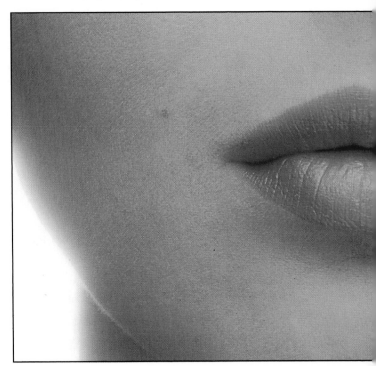

## Lip shapes and color

Examine your lips in a magnifying mirror in natural light. Do not wear lipstick, as you want to study the natural shape of your lips. Are they too small or too full compared with the rest of your face? Do you have an extremely thin upper lip and a fleshy lower one? Are both lips very wide? Could your lips use a little extra definition and shape? Is one of your lips lighter than the other? Once you've arrived at an assessment, you can start using lip color to change or define the shape of your lips.

Expert application of lip color can dramatically alter the shape of your lips by making them look wider, narrower, fuller or more finely shaped. Lighter shades will help to de-emphasize large or wide lips, while deep reds, browns and purples can reshape and emphasize lips that are narrow, tiny or thin.

Lip color comes in tiny jars of gloss, and in pencils, lipsticks with built-in brush applicators, and retractable lipstick tubes. For maximum control, use a natural-haired lip brush to apply lipstick. When choosing lip colors, do not test them on the back of your hand, unless you absolutely have no choice. Instead, put your thumb and forefinger together, pressing them hard so that the two of them change color. They'll redden slightly, and this redness will approximate your natural lip color. This is the only sure way of selecting colors appropriate for your skin tone. Be sure to select a blusher and eyeshadow that is complementary to your lipstick. If, for instance, your eyeshadow is in purple, blue and rose tones, you want a lip color that is a lilac, rose, or blue-pink color. Although you may adore festive colors, like apple red or metallic bronze, they will look garish unless you use a complementary blusher and eyeshadow.

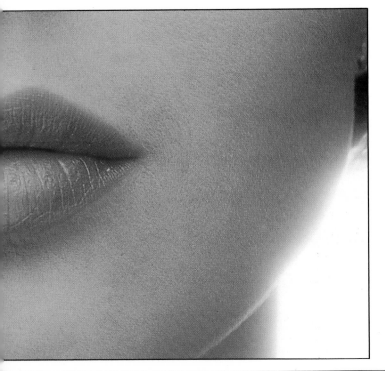

### Enhancing your normal lip definition

*If lipstick is applied alone, without a lip pencil outline, the resulting splash of color can make your lips look more imbalanced than they are. Use lip pencils for framing your lips to their best advantage. Remember that your lips should be dry when you apply lipstick.*

*1. Moisturize.*

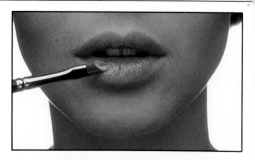

*2. To define normal lips, use your pencil to draw the outline in small, quick strokes, starting at the brow on the upper lip. This outline also helps to prevent lipstick from smearing. Continue the outline towards each corner of your mouth, keeping it closed and free of tension. Fill in the outline of the bottom lip and prepare the lip brush with color.*

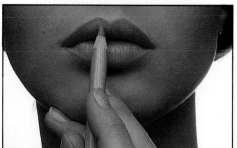

*3. Brush in color, starting at the center of your lip and working outwards; repeat on your lower lip.*

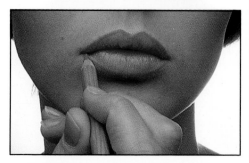

*4. Depending on the effect you want to achieve, smudge the pencil outline to blend with the lip color, or leave the outline half visible.*

*5. For extra shine, dab silver highlighter on the middle of your lower lip. Always blot lips with a tissue.*

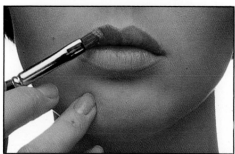

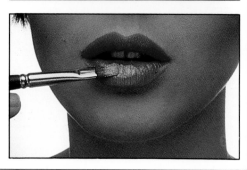

# MAKEUP TIPS FROM AN EXPERT

Patrick Dennis is an expert makeup artist who has been in the business for nine years. He is based in New York, although his work takes him all around the world. He has done features for several top European fashion magazines and his credits include the feature film, *The Tempest*, spreads in *Harper's Bazaar*, *Mademoiselle* and *Self*, and print and television advertisements for major cosmetic companies and fashion houses.

Patrick works only with liquid foundation, powdered eyeshadows, blushers, contour powder and powder. Because it is often difficult to control the intensity of liquid eye and cheek colors, he finds them impractical to use. Also liquid blushers and eyeshadows tend to change consistency according to temperature and humidity levels, so they are not as reliable as powdered cosmetics.

Patrick is very aware of the problems that Black and ethnically-mixed women have in trying to find make-up that blends well with darker, more exotic skin tones. He often resorts to mixing his own powders, blushers and contour powders for the models he is working with. You could try this too, if you're unhappy with the way your make-up goes with your skin tones. Blending yor own makeup colors can be time-consuming, but if you find the perfect shade of foundation, powder or eye color it will have been worth the effort.

For removing face makeup, Patrick Dennis suggests cleaning with cold cream and tissues, used one after the other, until the tissue wipes clean. Rinse your face in cool water, towel dry, and use an alcohol-free lotion toner on a cotton cosmetic pad for a final cleansing. If you have oily skin, use an alcohol based astringent. Remove eye makeup with baby oil and cotton cosmetic pads or, for sensitive eyes, use a hypo-allergenic lotion formulated for eye make-up removal. Women with very dry skins should try pure corn oil as a makeup remover. Use it in conjunction with cotton cosmetic pads; it is one of the cheapest and most effective cosmetics for dry-skinned complexions.

Because a professional model wears a lot of makeup, her skin is constantly covered up. Patrick Dennis suggests a professional facial once a month to open pores and give a deep clean. He also suggests that as little makeup as possible is worn when a model is not working. On days off, simply wear moisturizer and allow the skin to breathe.

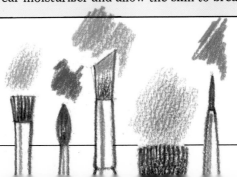

### How to make small lips look larger

*First, select a lip color and a lip pencil that is a shade darker for outlining. Define the bow part on your upper lip with the pencil in two precise, even strokes. Depending on how much you want to enlarge the lips, follow the line of the bow directly above the upper lip. Continue to outline towards the corner. Keep your mouth closed and relaxed. Always use precise, short strokes of the pencil; do not attempt to draw in a continuous line. Repeat with the lower lip, starting at the centre and working outwards, towards the corners. For maximum subtlety, gently smudge the pencil outline towards the inside of your lips. Now, take some color on to your lip brush and color in the outline with careful, short strokes. Start at the center of your mouth and work towards the corners, filling the lip area with color.*

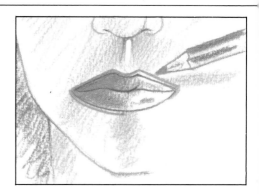

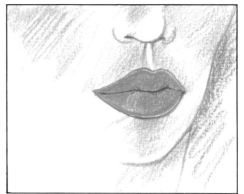

### How to minimize wide lips

*Outline your lips with a dark-toned lip pencil and fill in with matching, but slightly lighter, lipstick color. Smudge the outline so it blends a little with the lipstick. You want to avoid an exceptionally shiny or bright lipstick, as it will give the illusion of large lips. Stick with matt colors, and never wear lip gloss.*

### How to minimize full lips

*Outline just within the outer edge of your lips with a lip pencil. Start at the bow on the upper lip and stroke down towards each corner. Fill in the lower rim of the lip outline. Put some color that is a shade lighter than the pencil on to the lip brush and fill in your lips, starting at the center and working out to the corners. The best colors to use to minimize the size of your lips are a light pink or apricot-pink.*

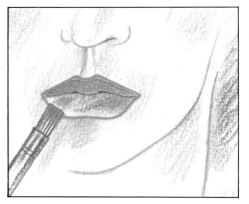

### How to balance a thin upper lip and a full lower lip

*Draw an outline beyond the outer edge of your upper lip with lip pencil to balance the proportions of the lips. Start above the bow on the upper lip and pencil in quick, small strokes. Brush on lip color, working gradually towards the outline in short, controlled strokes. Next, line the lower lip with pencil around the edge. Be sure to blend lip color starting from the center and working to the corner of the mouth.*

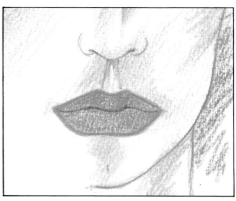

# Makeup care

Unless regularly sharpened, eye pencils build up a layer of oil and breed bacteria. Oil build-up results from the pencil's contact with the eyelid and inner rim of the eye and this can greatly reduce the color intensity of the makeup. To get the most out of your eye pencils, sharpen them regularly with pencil sharpeners — a metal one works best. Replace all of your eye pencils every four to six months — this will safeguard against eye infections. If you're a model, you'll probably need to replace mascara once a month, or every six weeks. Otherwise you should replace mascara every six months. Cake and powdered eyeshadow, if used only with cotton swabs, can remain relatively germ-free for up to a year.

You may have found that the texture of lipsticks and lip glosses grows drier after several months, causing irregular distribution of lip color or caking upon application. There is nothing you can do to lipsticks when they reach this stage, but to make your lip gloss last longer, mix in a dab of petroleum jelly, and it will spread evenly again. All other cosmetics, such as liquid foundation, powders and blushers, will keep for quite some time, but look for any changes in consistency or discoloration, and replace them with new products if necessary.

Regarding the removal of nail polish, use an acetone-free remover as acetone is a toxic substance and can be absorbed through the skin into the bloodstream.

It is a good idea to clean and replace brushes regularly to avoid the build-up of bacteria. Any woman who is prone to irritations and infections should follow this rule, instead of using the same eyeshadow brush day after day. It's a good idea to wash out your brushes every other week with lukewarm water and a heavily diluted, mild liquid detergent. The sponges that you use to apply your foundation should be rinsed out with lukewarm water once a week, and replaced every three months. Powder puffs and pads should be replaced as soon as a heavy build-up of color is visible, usually every six weeks or so. If you're a working model who regularly does her own make-up for shoots, then you should probably wash your brushes out every night and replace your sponges once or twice a week; always carry cotton swabs with you in your work bag, and replace powder pads once or twice a week, as necessary.

*First apply one coat of lipstick (a lipbrush will give greater accuracy), blot your lips, then apply another coat. This makes it last longer.*

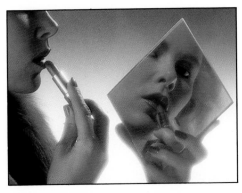

# HAIR CARE

Hair is the 'crowning glory' of your appearance and it can easily be your most striking asset. Nothing is more attractive than a shining head of hair; nothing can make you look and feel more unkempt than hair that is untidy and in need of a wash. Hair should be cut and conditioned at regular intervals, particularly if you are a professional model, as this will ensure maximum versatility for photographs.

Consider the following: every visible hair on your head is completely dead. Only the hair root under the scalp and inside the follicle is alive. Because your hair is essentially a mass of dead cells, it is impossible to change the permanent condition of it. Thus, because your hair tends to mirror the quality of your health, the best hair conditioner is a varied, well-balanced diet. To keep your hair in tip-top condition, you must first assess its basic nature and then care for it appropriately. If you have a serious hair problem — if you are going prematurely bald or your hair is falling out in patches — consult a trichologist, a doctor who specializes in treating hair disorders.

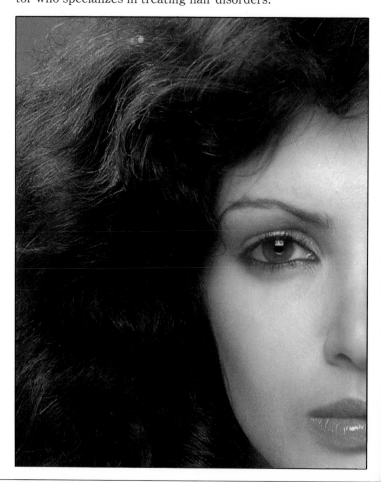

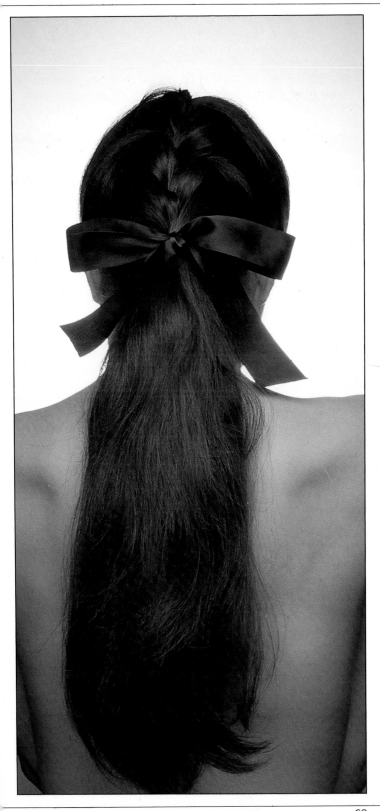

## Individual hair care

There are several basic hair types. Fine or flyaway hair, which does not hold a set and often looks limp. Thick hair which is quite resilient and, once set, holds shape for a day or more. Curly or wiry hair can be any texture — fine, thick or medium — and is often coarse. Medium-textured hair can be either naturally wavy or straight, and it can be styled in a variety of ways. It also sets very well.

You must base your hair-care program on the relative dryness, coarseness, frizziness or oiliness of your hair. Your selection of shampoos and conditioners and styling preparations is very important, as are frequent haircuts. According to Randy Davis, a versatile hair stylist at one of New York's top salons, 'no matter what the problem is with your hair, you can improve it by having frequent cuts or trims. There are also dozens of specially formulated hair-care products on the market today, and once you find the right ones for your hair, they can really help you to control it. Above all, diet is very important, and if you crash-diet, you can drastically weaken and dull the hair.'

A common mistake with hair care is the over-conditioning of fine, non-oily hair. Unless your hair is quite dry, never use products for dry hair on fine hair. Shampoos and conditioners formulated for fine hair will work better for your needs. Another frequent mistake is using products designed for oily hair or normal hair. To avoid this, choose shampoos that have pH5 (a balance of acid and alkaline). This represents the estimated normal acidity of the scalp, and will help to clean all hair types gently and effectively. When shampooing and conditioning, always rinse with lukewarm water, or colder water if you can stand it, as this will bring out the shine in your hair.

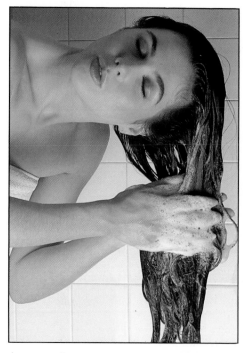

*No matter what your hair type, choose a shampoo that has a pH5 (a balance of acid and alkaline). This represents the normal acidity of the scalp and helps to clean all hair types gently and effectively. When shampooing and conditioning, always rinse with lukewarm water (or cold if you can bear it) to bring out the shine.*

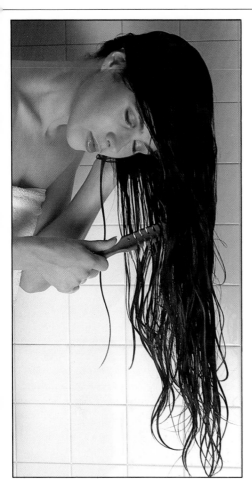

*Never brush your hair when wet. For safe untangling, always use a wide-tooth comb. Take a small section of hair and gently comb it through to the ends. Work slowly up to the top of your head, taking care not to pull or tug knots of hair as you go.*

## Conditioners

Conditioners are used after shampooing. If your hair is coarse or dry, fine or flyaway, you may want to condition it every time you shampoo to give your hair some smooth body and shine. If you regularly use either a blow dryer, electric curlers or a curling iron, you may find that your hair becomes so dry that you need daily conditioning, plus once-a-week deep-conditioning treatments. For a high-quality, outstanding weekly conditioner, try olive oil. Hair stylists and models recommend it for conditioning and brightening blond, light brown and red hair. To apply, massage oil into the scalp and out to the ends of your hair until your whole head is covered. Wrap your head in a thin towel or a cotton scarf and let the oil set for an hour or more. For maximum effect, leave it on overnight. In the morning, shampoo and rinse repeatedly. The same method can be followed using coconut oil, which brings out beautiful highlights in black and dark brown hair.

The conditioning value of cream rinses is debatable. Although many women use them after shampooing to untangle their hair and give it more bounce, most hair stylists seem to feel that you're better off using a hair conditioner.

## Styling preparations

There is now a wide range of preparations to choose from for controlling and styling your hair. These run the gamut from old-fashioned slick hair gels, to conditioning hair creams and aerosol-spray styling mousse. (The latter looks and feels like whipped cream yet handles wonderfully. It is particularly useful for a short, above-the-shoulders haircut.) Whether your hair is straight or curly, these preparations hold it in place while adding shine and shape to your hair.

For instance, if you have wavy or straight hair that reaches no further than the middle of your neck, try slicking your damp hair straight back (without a parting) for a dramatic, evening hairstyle. A thin coating of gel is best for this purpose; rub it into your palms with your fingertips before applying. If your hair is curly, try smoothing a small amount of gel, cream or mousse over your head and then run your fingers through the curls to hold them in a shiny, shapely set. You can also experiment with pump hair sprays — some of these are highly conditioned with protein and set a style as well as a gel can.

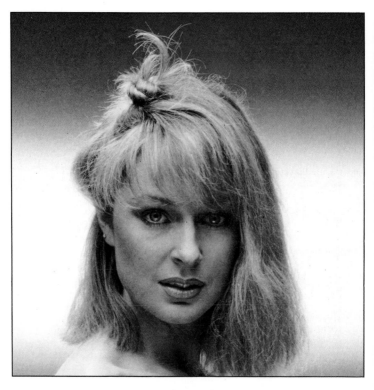

**Topknot** *Because of its versatility a medium-length bob is particularly good for models, who must be able to style their hair in many different ways. For a slightly different topknot, take a section of hair from the side of your head, twist it around and secure it with a pin or clip.*

**French Pleat** *For this pleat, bend your head forward. Take two sections of hair from the nape of your neck and twist one over the other. Twist again and add more hair from the opposite side of your head. Continue braiding, advancing from the nape of your neck to the top of your head.*

**Fishtail Plait** *For this inverted plait, take two sections of hair and twist one over the other. Add in extra hair from one side, then twist and add in hair from the other. Keep braid close to your head until you approach the nape of your neck, then begin a regular braid. Secure plait with a rubber band. For an unusual finish take a little hair from the front of your head, twist it and run a clip through it so that the hair splays out like a fan.*

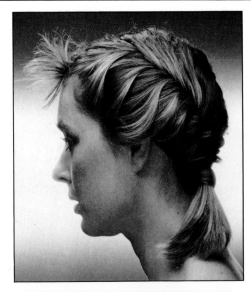

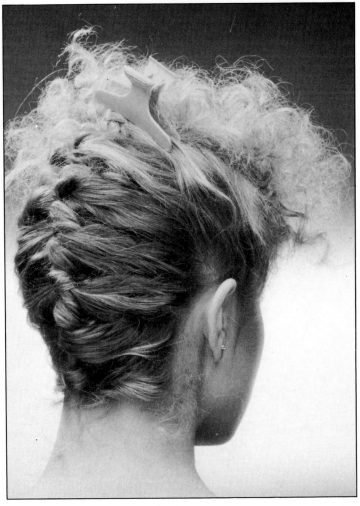

## Special products for problem hair

Common hair problems are dandruff, damaged hair that has been overdyed or overtreated with chemical permanent solutions, and hair that has a permanently dull look to it. These conditions can be treated by using specially formulated shampoos and conditioners. For serious problems, consult a trichologist. For instance, dandruff may become so severe that only a doctor

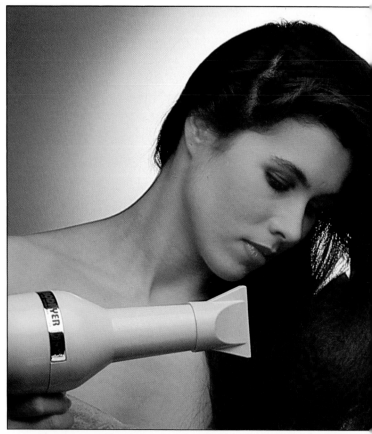

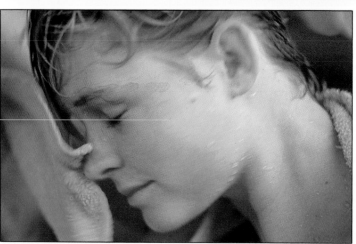

can relieve your symptoms. If your hair has been severely damaged by harsh hair dyes or permanent solutions, you may be wise just to cut off the damaged hair, and dye over the color in a darker shade. If your hair is quite dull and lifeless, this could reflect poor health or a nutritional deficiency. A trichologist could help you here by evaluating your diet and prescribing vitamin supplements accordingly.

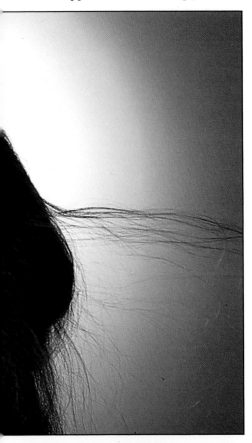

*With a hand-held blow-dryer, dry the hair around the head until it is damp. To style, take your comb and divide the top layers of your hair into two side sections and one at the back. Gently twist each side section, and pin on top of head. Dry hair underneath the back section first. Next, dry the sides, stretching the hair lightly with a round styling brush. Follow the brush strokes with the hair dryer. To curl the hair under, brush from underneath. For turned-up curls, place the brush on top to curl up and out. For more dramatic short-term styles, use electric tongs (below right) on dry hair.*

*Today's free unstructured hair styles allow you to put shape and movement into your hair simply by towel or finger-drying (below left).*

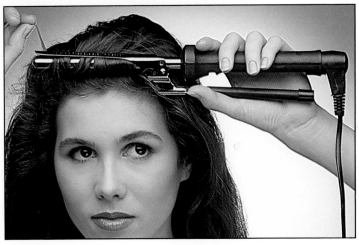

## Choosing a hairstyle

For the professional model, or any woman who wants a flexible hairstyle, the best cut is shoulder-length, and slightly layered around the face. This style gives you the freedom to wear the hair in several ways. You can also blow-dry it straight, or set it in waves with a fringe for framing the face. This classic cut requires weekly conditioning and a once-a-month trim. If you are looking for a hairstyle that is ideally flattering to your shape of face, then the following advice may be helpful.

## Straightening or relaxing your hair

Hair straighteners come in liquid form and chemically re-arrange the natural structure of curly hair into a straight configuration. Relaxers do the same thing, only their effect is more gentle, resulting in loose curls or waves. These preparations are usually fairly harsh and should not be used at home. Improper application can result in scalp burns, hair loss, frizzing, or dulling of hair colour. Consult an experienced hairdresser if you want your hair straightened or relaxed. Be sure to ask for instructions on how to condition your hair after having either hair treatment.

## Perming your hair

A 'permanent' curls your hair by breaking the chemical bonds that hold your hair in shape and altering them to form a pattern set by different-sized curlers on your head. A permanent *must* be administered by a professional, as you do not want to risk damaging your hair by misusing the chemical solutions or styling the curlers incorrectly. Ask your hairstylist to recommend the best conditioning formula for your hair, and remember to wait a day or two before shampooing newly permed hair.

**Hairstyles for very curly or wiry hair**
*An attractive and easily maintained look for this type of hair is a short, neat cut that is no longer than an inch all the way round. Style it with hair gel or cream and you've got classic, well-dressed curls. Long, angelic ringlets or a bushy Afro can also complement certain shapes of face. If you are Black, you may feel like trying a traditional African hairstyle, such as tiny, short braids patterned in rows, or long braids with beads strung in between the braids. This will emphasize your features as well as provide a naturally stylish look.*

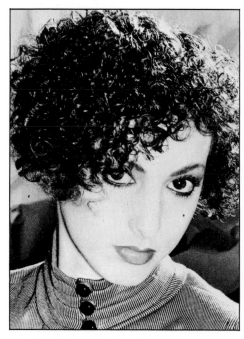

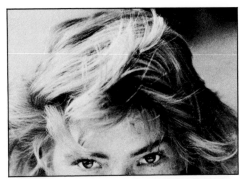

**Hairstyles for a large forehead**
A fringe is the easiest way to play down a large forehead. Round faces usually look rounder with a fringe, and long faces are somewhat shortened. Another cut that may work for your face shape is a shoulder-length, layered cut that is parted on the side and falls forward on your forehead.

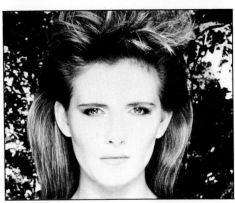

**Hairstyles for a round face**
Hair that is layered and falls to the shoulders or below is very attractive, as it shows your face, yet makes it look narrower than it really is. Short, side-parted blunt cuts that are about shoulder length are also recommended.

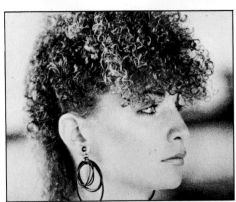

**Hairstyles for a heart-shaped face**
Shoulder-length, blunt-cut hair or wavy hair with a fringe looks best with this face shape. Depending on the size of your bones, however, you may decide that you want to wear your hair longer than shoulder length. Hair cut above the shoulder tends to emphasize the angles of a heart-shaped face, but if you're comfortable with a striking look, shorter hair may be for you.

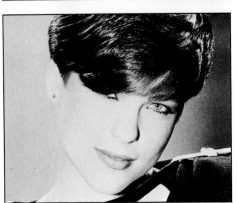

**Hairstyles for a long face**
The longer your hair is, the longer and more angular your face will look. To give your face a softer, rounder look, try a shoulder-length, slightly layered cut with a fringe. Close-cropped hair is always in fashion — if your neck is long enough and you're ready for a big change, try a very short style.

## Coloring your hair

Changing the color of your hair can be a risky business. Dyeing your hair can weaken it and make it brittle, and dyed hair should always be kept away from the sun unless you welcome green, red or purple highlights. It is also important to shampoo dyed hair immediately after leaving salt water or chlorine pools, otherwise you will acquire unsightly streaks. If you are contemplating a career as a professional model, stay with your natural shade rather than trying anything as irreversible as hair coloring. This also goes for bleaching, frosting and highlighting your hair. If you really desire to be a platinum blonde or redhead, then consult a professional hair colorist. He or she will be able to suggest the best shades and methods of changing your hair, and will be sure to match your hair color with your eyebrows and general skin tone.

## Accessories and styling

The most essential haircare accessory is a hairbrush — choose one with plastic bristles spaced far apart for basic hair grooming, as well as a round styling brush for straightening hair as you style it, or giving hair more waves. You may also want a wide-tooth comb for disentangling wet hair, and hair clips for sectioning your hair as you style it. A hand-held blow dryer is another essential tool for hair styling, unless you have a style that can be

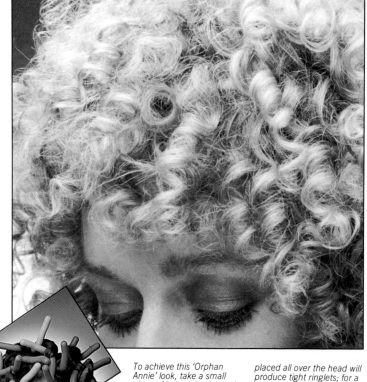

To achieve this 'Orphan Annie' look, take a small piece of hair and twist each piece twice, always in the same direction, and roll it onto a curler. Curlers placed all over the head will produce tight ringlets; for a slightly softer look, simply brush hair out to give loose curls.

rubbed dry. Here is the technique for basic blow-dry styling: set the dryer on the medium or cool setting, hold the dryer at least 6in (15cm) from your head, as high heat will damage your hair and dry it out within a few minutes. Dry the hair around the head until it is damp. Take your comb and start dividing the top layers of your hair into sections. Make two at each side and one at the back. Gently twist each section, except for the back, and pin firmly on top of the head. Dry the hair underneath the back section first. Next dry the sides, stretching the hair lightly with the brush, and following the brush strokes with the hair dryer. To curl the hair in or under, brush from underneath. For turned-up curls, use the brush above to curl up and out.

For more pronounced styling, you will want to set your hair with rollers or curlers. Most professional models use electric curlers, as they often need to change hairstyles several times a day for different fashion shows or photographs. Electric curlers do not hold a set for very long, but they can achieve dramatic, short-term results. Your hair should be totally dry when setting with electric curlers; most have plastic-tipped pins for anchoring them in place, so don't use metal ones as a substitute, as they can burn your scalp when used in conjunction with electric rollers. When the rollers have cooled, remove them.

To add body or achieve loose curls, use medium-sized rollers. Working upwards from your neckline, roll the hair at the sides and back from the root downwards. This will give you two side sections, and one front section, which are your bangs. You will have the maximum amount of waves if you have the slightly layered haircut suggested at the beginning of this section. Complete the set by rolling the central section of your bangs forward.

For a curlier set, roll the two sections at the nape of the neck downwards, on narrow rollers. For the middle layers, use six or seven narrow rollers placed vertically, not horizontally, like the previous setting instructions for loose curls. Roll this hair towards your face. With the top layers, make an asymmetrical or side part and roll the hair down on large rollers.

If you want a set that will last for some time, then you should use regular rollers, setting lotion and a wet head of hair. First apply a generous amount of setting lotion to your hair with a wide-tooth comb. Be sure to comb the lotion behind your ears. Now section your hair by parting and pinning it up on your head. For this kind of setting you will need endpapers (also called setting paper). These tiny strips should be folded over the ends of your hair as you curl; the rollers are placed over the papers and you should roll them slowly backward to the root of the hair. Clip the rollers to the roots with tiny hair clips. Your rollers should be anchored to your scalp, but not so tight that they are pulling your hair. Repeat this all over the head. The rollers should lie horizontally on the top and vertically at the sides. This will give your hair both waves and body.

To achieve tighter curls, follow the instructions previously given in this section for a curlier set. To hold your set, try misting your head with a fine spray of water, held 6in (15cm) away from the head.

# BODY CARE

Now that you have learned about the value of exercise, diet, facial care and makeup, the next step is to consider how to care for the rest of your body. Along with a daily skin-care routine, this is an integral part of the life of a model. The essentials that you need to know regarding sun-tanning, dental care, foot and hand care are all detailed in the following section.

## Ways to youthful skin

Showering, exercise, suntanning and cold weather can irritate your skin and cause it to peel, flake or itch. To relieve normal skin dryness, moisturize at least twice a day, or as needed, on pronounced dry spots. The most efficient moisturizers are creams that contain a balance of fatty acids and alcohols which are readily absorbed by the skin. When selecting a moisturizing cream, remember that it must be able to conserve the water in your skin. If it is thick and dense, it will only clog your pores.

Oils are also useful for moisturizing dry spots, but one disadvantage is that they are not as quickly absorbed by the skin as creams are. Because you need an overall body moisturizer, however, you should go ahead and experiment with both to find the right product for your particular skin type. If you have dry or sensitive skin, you should look for hypo-allergenic products. These will probably be more gentle on your skin.

## The sun and your skin

Although we absorb Vitamin D from sunlight through our skin, the sun's ultraviolet rays are unquestionably harmful to the skin's four layers. Unprotected and prolonged exposure to the sun can cause redness, inflammation, swelling or blistering, and the fairer your skin is the more damage can be done to it. The sun's rays force the skin to experience a deadening, malignant change that can encourage skin cancer. Another long-term effect of suntanning is loss of firmness and elasticity from the skin. This causes early wrinkles and has a physically ageing effect.

If you are considering suntanning salons or sunbeds as the quickest route to a deep suntan, then you should understand what the risks are. Suntanning salons frequently use ultra-violet light ray waves that are known to cause skin cancer, premature ageing and cataracts. Devices such as sun beds, which resemble giant-size waffle irons, are also potentially dangerous because of the quality of the light rays.

*Unprotected and prolonged exposure to the sun can cause redness, inflammation and blistering. So if you have fair skin, choose a sunscreen lotion with a high Sun Protection Factor.*

## Protection from sunburn

Although most dermatologists agree that sunbathing can prematurely age and otherwise damage the skin, if you decide to suntan, there are protective measures that you can, and should, take. There are sunscreen lotions and creams on the market that prevent the skin from burning, and some can even prevent tanning altogether. Look for products that state their Sun Protection Factor (SPF) on the label. An SPF of 20 means that you can sun up to 20 times longer than you could without protection. On most people, sunscreens with an SPF of 20 prevent tanning. Sunscreens with SPF 15 are a good choice for fair-skinned people who cannot risk burning yet desire a slight suntan. Medium skins should stick between the SPF ranges of 3 to 15, depending on how easily you tend to burn and how dark you'd like your suntan to be.

Because the sun dries your skin and causes peeling, you must moisturize your face and body after all suntanning sessions. This will nourish your skin and reduce future peeling. Moisturizers with natural oils such as aloe, coconut, avocado and almond are the best lubricants for slightly reddened or tanned skins.

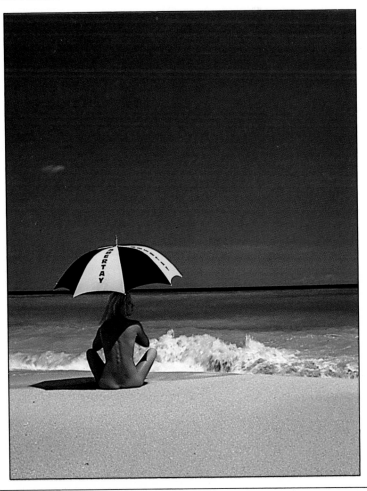

## Hair removal

Excessive body hair or facial hair can be very unattractive. Certainly, a model will not be regarded as a professional if her photographs show hints of either. Both body hair and facial hair must be removed, and in the case of a model it is advisable to remove hair permanently.

The most popular method of permanent hair removal is electrolysis, which destroys the root of the hair by chemical reaction. If you are looking for an electrolysist, try to find one who is professionally licensed and who has treated someone you know. On your first visit, make sure that the operator tests a small patch of skin to discover your sensitivity to this process before treating a large area. A word of warning: never try to remove hair from the inside upper thighs with electrolysis. The best method for a 'bikini shave' is to use a razor and shaving cream. If the hairs are long, first cut them as short as you can with scissors, and then shave slowly and carefully. Remember that electrolysis treatment can be painful and is fairly costly.

For women who are not interested in permanent hair removal, there are other methods available that may suit their particular needs. For the temporary removal of facial hair on the upper lip and elsewhere, for example, cream depilatory is quite popular and effective. This dissolves the hair and gives smoother, longer-lasting results than shaving. Some people may be allergic to the chemical ingredients in depilatory cream so be sure to test a small patch of skin (try your forearm) with the depilatory before applying it to your face. An alternative way of dealing with facial hair is to use cosmetic bleach — you can buy this from any pharmacy and it will effectively lighten the hair so that it is less noticeable.

For the removal of heavy underarm or leg hair, many women choose to have hot wax treatments. The method is simple, but if the wax is not heated to the correct temperature and coated thinly across the skin area, the removal process can be very painful. When applied correctly the wax is cooled slightly and then ripped off in strips, pulling the hairs out by their roots. Waxing results in very soft and smooth skin, and the hair takes longer to grow back than with any other temporary removal method. Waxing is recommended for the face, legs, arms, underarms and inside upper thighs.

*An ordinary wet shaver can be used to remove underarm hair, but always apply shaving cream first.*

*An electric shaver can also be used to remove underarm hair quickly and is gentler than a wet shave.*

*This spray-on depilatory cream is another, longer-lasting method of temporary hair removal that gives a smoother finish than shaving.*

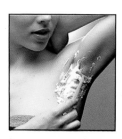
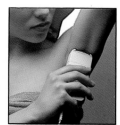
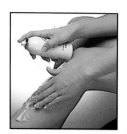

# DENTAL CARE

If you follow a daily routine of proper brushing and flossing and see your dentist regularly, you should have no problems with your teeth. However, proper care of your teeth also involves caring for your gums. Brushing and flossing after every meal can keep both teeth and gums in top shape. Choose a toothbrush that is flat on top and has tightly packed bristles — nylon bristles are considered more effective than natural ones, as they have a uniform shape and will clean more effectively. The bristles should be semi-soft and able to reach the gums without causing undue bleeding or pain. Your toothbrush should be replaced once the bristles start to lose their shape, usually after about three months. If you have to replace your brush more often than this you are probably brushing too hard. Here's how to brush properly: start at the back of the mouth, on the outer side of your lower jaw. Hold the brush so that it is at a 45-degree angle to the gum. It must lie lengthwise across the teeth as the bristles must be able to clean the area where the gum meets the tooth. With a light touch move the bristles back and forth 20 times and do the same on all the other areas around the jaw. Repeat this method on the inner surface of the tooth on the lower jaw. Then brush the top of the teeth on your lower jaw. Now brush your upper jaw in the same way, brushing both the inside and outside of your teeth. Finally, rinse your mouth out with cold water.

No matter how carefully you brush your teeth every day, the combination of a fluoride toothpaste and a semi-soft toothbrush will clean only three of the five sides of the teeth. Particles of food get trapped between the teeth, breeding bacteria that attacks the gums and surrounding bone. The only way you can clean the spaces between your teeth is by thorough flossing before every brushing. Dental floss comes in waxed and unwaxed forms. Dr Leonard Sklar, a New York oral surgeon, recommends the unwaxed variety because it is less irritating to the gums. To use floss, break off about a foot-long strip and hold it between the thumb and index finger of both hands. Wrap floss around the tooth in a wide V — almost a boomerang shape. Now slide the floss down so that it touches the gum and bring it up again. Do this six times if you are flossing daily, more if you are not, and change the direction of the floss so that you are cleaning the surface of the adjacent tooth.

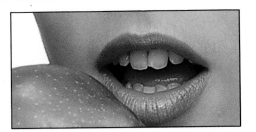

*Heathy teeth and gums are sure signs of wellbeing and will enhance your appearance every time you smile. Crisp fruit and raw vegetables are good for teeth, but they are no substitute for careful brushing and flossing.*

# HAND CARE

Soap and water, cold and hot air, detergents, harsh chemicals and numerous other irritants all take their toll on your hands. Because hands receive such a beating, it's important to take good care of them, properly cleaning and moisturizing them daily. When washing your hands, use a moisturizing soap and rinse several times. Dry your hands thoroughly and apply either your overall body moisturizer or an effective hand cream. If your hands are dry, always carry a tube of cream with you in your purse to soothe your skin and prevent further dryness. In extreme cases, chapping can lead to eczema, which should be treated by a doctor. To protect hands, wear plastic gloves while washing dishes or clothes but do not wear them for more than 10-15 minutes at a time. If your palms tend to perspire, a weak solution of aluminum chloride and water, applied with a cotton cosmetic pad, will help them cool down and dry out naturally.

### Nail care

Split and broken nails are a common problem that affects hands and can detract from their appearance. There is a popular theory that gelatine helps build strong, healthy nails, but this is a myth. The only way you can nourish your nails is to eat well — an imbalanced diet can cause nails to crack or break — and treat them with a weekly home manicure. Remember when applying nail polish that all polish (base, polish, sealer) is applied three strokes to the nail. Start at the base of your nail and finish at the nail's end. The first stroke is down the center of your nail. The second and third strokes are on either side of the first one. Occasionally, the nail plate will separate from the nail bed because of excessive use of nail hardeners. This can cause infection and discoloration. Should this occur, trim the nail very short. To keep nails flexible and prevent painful hang nails, moisturize with cold cream every night.

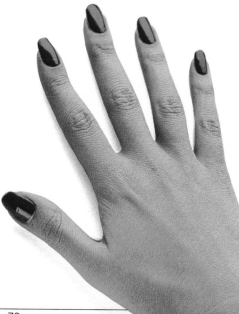

Despite the harsh treatment they come in for, hands are one of the most neglected parts of the body. Very few women meet the requirements for a professional hand model: strong hands (hand modelling can be tiring) with long, slender fingers, tapered fingertips, narrow palms, and immaculately manicured nails. To keep their hands beautiful and preserve them from any damage, many hand models are careful to always wear gloves.

Even if you don't have the long slender fingers of the professional hand model, you should keep your hands in flawless condition. Apply daily a hand cream or moisturizer, protect your hands from water and harsh weather by wearing gloves, keep nails well-trimmed and have frequent manicures.

A manicure once every two weeks is essential to keep your hands in tip-top condition. Women who work with their hands or whose hands are subjected to harsh chemicals or frequent wetting may need a manicure once a week.

## Equipment checklist

Assemble the following: cotton wool, nail-polish remover, an emery board, petroleum jelly, baby oil, moisturizer, a soft toothbrush, and an orange stick.

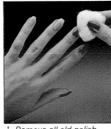
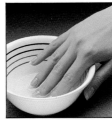

1. Remove all old polish with cotton cosmetic pads and nail-polish remover. Do not soak your nails before filing, as this will make them break easier.

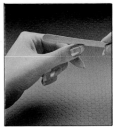
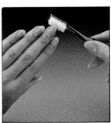

2. File each nail with an emery board by gently stroking from the side to the center do not file back and forth.

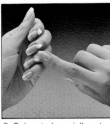

3. Rub petroleum jelly onto all of your cuticles and apply moisturizing cream to your nails and hands.

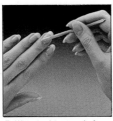

4. Now, warm three-quarters of a cup of baby oil on the stove. Do not boil. Pour into a small bowl and soak your fingertips in the oil for five minutes.

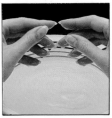

5. With a soft toothbrush, remove any matter from underneath your nails. Rinse your hands under warm water and dry off thoroughly.

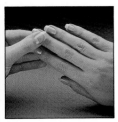

6. Using your fingertips, train your cuticles back.

7. With the blunt end of an orange stick, train the cuticles back again. Never try to cut your cuticles.

8. Rinse your hands again in warm water and remove any traces of baby oil. Your manicure is now complete. If you are going to apply polish to your nails, you should wait five minutes.

There are a few key steps to follow when applying nail polish. Always apply a base to your nails first. This will protect them from being stained by the polish. Let the base dry for five absorbent cotton, nail-polish bottle between your two palms. Do not shake it. Open the bottle and gently dip the brush in and out to gather enough polish for three nail strokes, applying the first stroke to the centre, the other two to the sides. Let the polish dry for 10 minutes and repeat with a second coat. After waiting 10 minutes, apply sealer to your nails and let dry for 20-30 minutes.

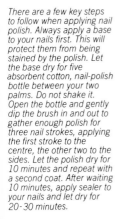
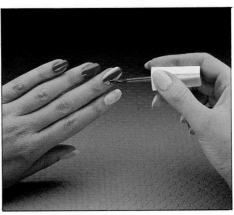

# FOOT CARE

Probably no part of the human body is as abused as our feet — they must bear our weight every day, carry us miles (the average person will walk the equivalent of three times around the world in a lifetime), and endure constriction in cramped, tight-fitting shoes.

It is not surprising, then, that many of us suffer from minor foot problems such as bunions, corns and verrucas. Models are especially vulnerable as they spend long days posing and parading up and down in high heels. Accordingly, a few words on the prevention and treatment of foot problems are appropriate here.

Bunions are inflamed thickenings on the underside of the big toe. They can be soothed by placing a padding inside the shoe with specially designed toe cushions. If bunions become too painful you should have them surgically removed.

Corns are thick pads of hardened skin that form on the toes and soles of the feet as a result of friction and tight-fitting shoes. Although corns are difficult to prevent, you can treat them with a corn plaster, or have them professionally treated by a foot specialist.

A verruca is an ingrowing wart on the foot caused by a common virus. Like all warts, it is infectious. Do not bathe in public swimming pools or showers if you have one and consult a dermatologist immediately for treatment. Never try to remove a verruca yourself; you risk scarring yourself and spreading the infection.

An ingrown toenail is a toenail that grows in a curved direction and digs into the skin at the side of your toe. Ingrown toenails can be exceedingly painful, and since the shape of your toes is genetically determined, you can do nothing to prevent your nails from growing sideways and inwards. What you can do, however, is avoid all tight shoes and socks. When cutting your toe nails, always trim straight across, leaving enough nail to cover the tip of the toe.

## FOOT PROBLEMS

*Foot problems are usually self-inflicted. The best way to prevent them is to wear comfortable, well-fitting shoes, not the platform soles, stiletto heels or pointed shoes that may happen to be in fashion. Keep these points in mind when buying shoes:*

*1. Any shoe you buy should be ½in (1cm) longer than your foot and should provide plenty of room for you to wriggle your toes.*
*2. Shoes must fit perfectly round the heels.*
*3. Shoes should not pinch, rub and squeeze any part of the foot and should provide plenty of support for your arch. Never buy a tight-fitting shoe and expect it to 'give'.*

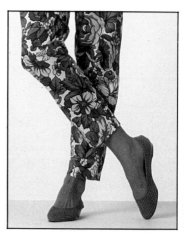

To forestall foot troubles and keep your feet looking attractive, give yourself a pedicure once every two weeks. If you happen to walk or exercise a great deal, you may need one every week. Just as before a manicure, remove all traces of polish from your toes.

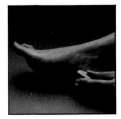

*1. Wash each foot in turn in soapy water, but do not soak feet.*

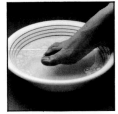

*2. With a pumice stone, gently rub the soles and heels to shed hard skin.*

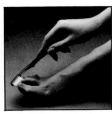

*3. Use a soft toothbrush to remove debris from underneath and around the nails.*

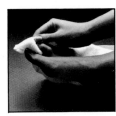

*4. Dry your feet thoroughly, especially between your toes.*

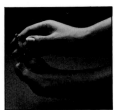

*5. Always trim the nails with a toenail clipper or nail scissors, cutting straight across. Leave nails long enough to cover the tip of the toe.*

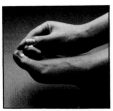

*6. Apply petroleum jelly to the base and sides of the nails with your fingertips.*

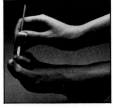

*7. With the blunt end of an orange stick, work at the base and sides of your nails to gradually ease the skin back. Be very gentle near the base of your nail. Let the jelly sit and condition for five minutes and then remove with cotton cosmetic pads.*

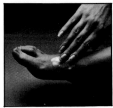

*8. Finally rub some moisturizer onto the top and bottom of your feet and onto your toes.*

To round off your pedicure, apply a touch of nail varnish. Avoid chipped, peeling nail varnish by applying one layer of base coat to clean nails, followed by two layers of colour. Allow each layer to dry thoroughly.

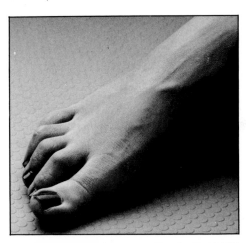

# 3

# FIRST IMPRESSIONS

## POSTURE

## DRESS SENSE

## THE RIGHT ATTITUDE

## ACCESSORIES

*T*he impression that you make on others at social gatherings, job interviews or in office situations, is decisively molded by your attitude and the way in which you present yourself. Subtle indicators of attitude include body language, carriage, the way you wear your clothes and the pitch and tempo of your voice. Although you may think that you can easily mask feelings of insecurity, anxiety or boredom, people can usually sense your mood. Self-assurance comes from walking with a natural air of confidence, holding yourself well and knowing that your appearance is right.

# POSTURE

Your posture is a signal to others of your personality and feelings. When you sit, stand, walk or dance, your body language communicates your energy, health and moods. Whether you are slim and fit, or overweight and out of shape, bad posture is a negative signal. It not only makes you look heavier than you are, it gives a very poor first impression. Improving your posture can take a considerable strain off your back, relieve muscular tension and make you look more erect and self-confident.

An excellent solution for anyone with bad posture is to study dance. Many women, including successful models, owe their elegant carriage to jazz, ballet or modern dance lessons. A good dance class will help you to increase your muscular flexibility while improving your balance. The primary benefit of regular dance classes is that they make the student aware of breathing and movement in a way that no other disciplined exercise can. They are more beneficial than old-fashioned deportment classes, because in dance, every part of the body is stretched and movements must be controlled and balanced.

Poise is not learned simply by walking along a straight line, with books balanced on top of your head. To understand what is wrong with your posture, you'll need a full-length mirror with good quality glass that is free of distortion. Spend some time studying yourself in the mirror so that you can see the shape and stance of your body. Now stand correctly with both feet on the floor and your legs

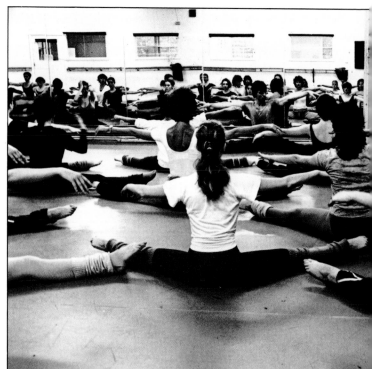

First impressions are important. Self-assurance comes from wearing smart clothes you feel comfortable in, walking with a natural air of confidence, and good posture.

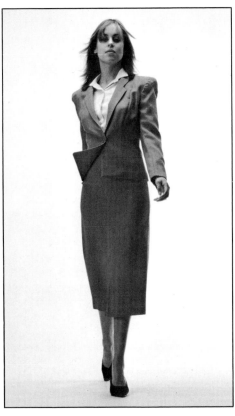

In addition to improving your posture and balance, attending a good dance class will help you to increase your muscular flexibility.

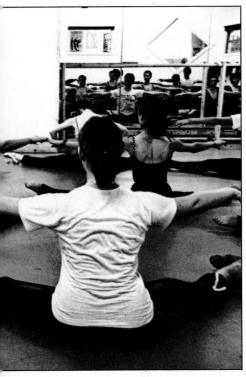

straight. Let your arms hang comfortably at your sides, elbows slightly bent. Hold your head straight, with your chin parallel to the floor — your shoulders should be level and relaxed. Hold your stomach in (do not overtense your muscles) and your rib cage high. You should also hold your buttocks in. Study yourself in this position for a moment and then relax into your normal standing position. You will immediately notice the difference — perhaps your shoulders are slumped or uneven, or your head is lowered.

## Walking tall

As any professional model, fashion photographer or modeling agent will tell you, your posture and the way that you walk tell volumes about your self-confidence. Knowing how to walk correctly, whether in the office or on a fashion-show catwalk, definitely increases your ability to make a winning first impression. Another indispensable tool for creating a positive response is the cultivation of your own personal style. This means learning how to coordinate outfits that flatter your figure, for even the most graceful walk in the world cannot disguise a lack of dress sense.

Before you begin scrutinizing your wardrobe, you must first examine the way that you walk. Look at the shoes that you wear most often and check the soles and the heels. If they look worn down unevenly on either side, then your walk needs attention. If you walk correctly, your posture will mirror the way you look when standing still, and your shoes will be evenly worn on the heels or soles. When you walk, let your arms swing naturally, but not in a jaunty or aggressive motion, and make sure that your weight is evenly distributed as you move. As your arm moves forward, your leg should go back.

You can perfect your walk by practicing for 15 minutes each day, concentrating on training your body to move in well-measured, natural steps. Simply lay down a thick strip of masking tape in a straight line (at least 2ft/36cm long) across a bare floor. Always practise walking without shoes, in your bare feet. With your first step, place the inside edge of your right foot to the right side of the line, barely touching it. Now step with your left foot forward and plant it to the left of the line, also barely grazing it. Walk slowly down the masking-tape line with your head erect and your eyes looking straight ahead. Neither foot should cross the line, and both feet should always fall at nearly the same distance from either side of the line. Never look down as you walk — only look to check the position of your feet once you come to the end of the line.

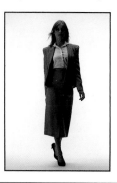
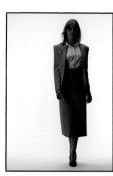

*Evaluate your stride. Is it erect and as fluid as it can be?*

How does your body and posture compare with this model's stance?

Always hold your head up straight, chin up. Your back and shoulders should be evenly set, erect and re-laxed. This will keep your chest aligned with the rest of your body. Keep stomach and buttocks tucked in to streamline your silhouette. Distribute your weight evenly on both feet for maximum balance and poise.

If you are slightly overweight, this will affect your carriage negatively. Bear in mind that you can easily correct your figure through diet, exercise, and commitment.

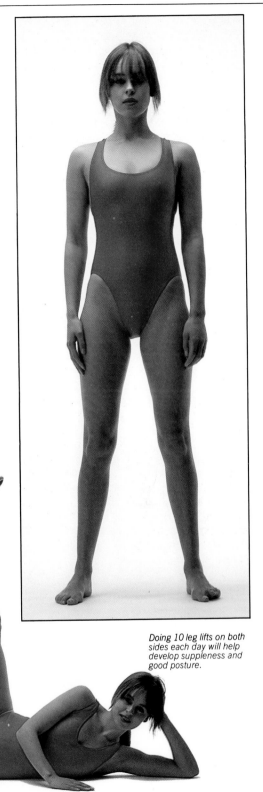

Doing 10 leg lifts on both sides each day will help develop suppleness and good posture.

**How to straighten your back and shoulders.** The two most common posture problems seem to be rounded shoulders and crooked backs. As mentioned before, these conditions can be improved by disciplined dance study. Ballet is known to be extremely effective in correcting back, shoulder and neck problems, but there are also exercises that you can do at home to help straighten your body. Try the following exercises and you'll see a difference in a week or two. In addition to improving your posture, these exercises can also be used to relieve backache and menstrual pain.

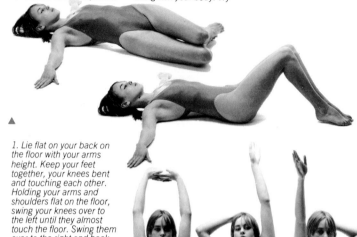

1. Lie flat on your back on the floor with your arms height. Keep your feet together, your knees bent and touching each other. Holding your arms and shoulders flat on the floor, swing your knees over to the left until they almost touch the floor. Swing them over to the right and back again. Repeat 15 times.

2. Another limbering-up exercise for you to try is this very simple rope climb. Stand with feet shoulder-width apart and stretch both arms upwards, clasping them above your head with palms facing up. Unlock your hands and reach up as far as possible, first with your right hand and then with your left, as if you were climbing a rope. Keep your feet firmly on the floor as you do this, as the idea is to stretch your back and shoulders as much as possible. Continuing the climbing arm movements, slowly bend forward from the waist, reaching towards the floor. When your hands are almost touching the floor, hold for five seconds and feel the stretch in your back and shoulders. Then work slowly back up until you are in your original position. Repeat 15 times. If you feel strained at any point, stop immediately. If you can carry on for 15 minutes without discomfort, then try to do this two or more times each day. The more you do this exercise, the more likely you are to improve your posture.

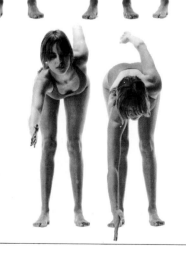

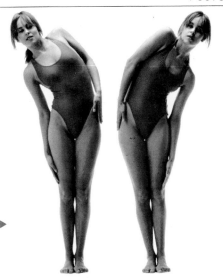

3. To straighten your shoulders, stand with legs together, head erect and back straight. Raise your right shoulder up towards your ear, and then slowly roll it backwards in the largest circle you can make. Reverse the rotation and repeat 15 times. Switch to your left shoulder for 15 repetitions and rest for 10 seconds. Now move both shoulders in a backward circular motion 10 times. If your shoulders are noticeably rounded, then do this exercise both in the morning and at night. After a full week, you'll be limber enough to do it in your lunch hour or breaks during the day.

4. This advanced back and shoulder exercise should only be done after you have mastered the previous three. Stand with your feet apart, at shoulder-width, knees slightly bent. Bend sideways from your hips and let your left arm hang comfortably at your side. Swing your right arm to the left as far as it will go, then bring it down and around to the right so that your hand hovers above the floor. Continuing the same motion, sweep your arm up to the right as high as you can. Your head should follow the movement of your arm during this exercise. Slowly swing back to your original position and repeat 10 times.

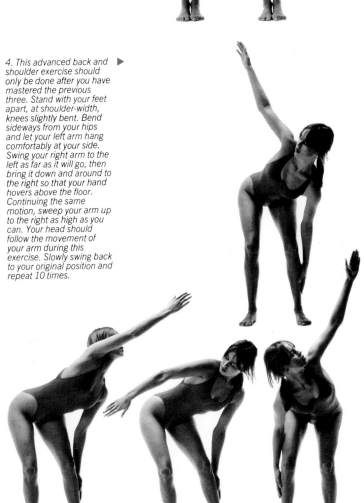

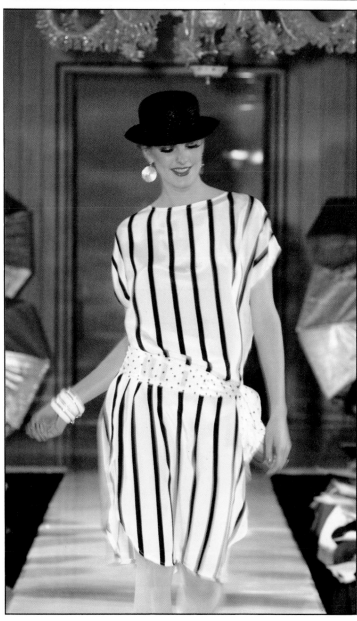

The fashion model on the catwalk (above) have learned the art of walking gracefully. Practice your own walk 15 minutes each day. Lay down a thick strip of masking tape in a straight line across a bare floor. Place the inside edge of your right foot to the right side of the line, barely grazing it. Now place your left foot to the left of the line. Slowly walk like this down the masking-tape line, with head erect and eyes looking straight ahead.

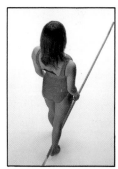

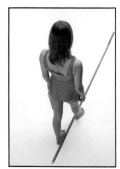

*Sitting correctly is an essential component of good posture as well as good health. Slouching (far right) can impede breathing; crossing your legs causes unnecessary muscular tension, slows down circulation and aggravates varicose veins. When sitting correctly (right) your shoulders should be square, your back straight, your rib cage high and your stomach held in. Your weight should be supported by the bones you are sitting on and your legs should be together on the floor.*

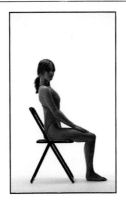
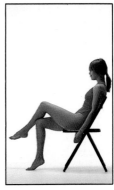

## Sitting pretty

Good body alignment and posture is essential to any modeling career, and it is also vital to your health. Slumped shoulders can put pressure on your chest and lungs and prevent you from breathing properly. Moreover, unlikely as it sounds, slouching can cause life-long digestive problems. These are just some of the reasons why sitting correctly is another essential component of good posture and natural poise.

Before you sit down, stand with your back to the chair, head up. Lower yourself into the chair slowly and smoothly. When you are seated, your back should be straight, your stomach should be held in and your rib cage should be high. Your weight should be supported by the bones you are sitting on, not by your thighs. Your legs should be together at all times — crossing them can slow down the circulation and aggravate varicose veins, as well as cause unnecessary muscular tension.

## Movement and poise

The most efficient way to master the art of moving and walking like a professional model is by going to live fashion shows at department stores, manufacturer's showrooms and, if possible, designers' salons. You will learn invaluable lessons by watching, criticizing, and copying the movements made by models. Observing others will enable you to study your own movements and will help you to discover how to express the appropriate mood for the clothes that you are wearing. Practise at home in a variety of outfits, especially heavy, layered winter clothing. If you can appear to move effortlessly in bulky sweaters, hats, boots and a winter coat, then you have learned a vitally important modeling skill. You would be well advised to practice in high heels as well as flat shoes, as these are the most difficult to walk in and are required for most modeling assignments. If you can walk gracefully in stiletto-heeled and open-toed sandals, then you will move gracefully in any kind of shoe or boot. The key to this is practice. Do not be discouraged if you look stiff or ungainly; take things gradually, and do not be impatient. Ask one of your friends to watch you as you practice — an objective observer can be very helpful in pointing out flaws and telling you when you have developed a graceful style. The most important factor is self-confidence — try to project this as you walk down the street or go through your practice routines.

# DRESS SENSE

Chapters One and Two showed how the way that you feel can affect the way that you look. Where clothing is concerned, however, you must be aware that the style and look of your outfit invariably influence how others perceive you. Clothing is an unspoken language, charged with subtle, impressive powers that words do not possess. Psychological surveys have proved that prospective employers are most impressed with those applicants (no matter what their actual qualifications are) who dress in fastidiously neat, traditional clothing and accessories. An excellent way to enhance your businesslike demeanor, whether you're being interviewed for a junior position or an executive one, is to carry a classic dark-brown or black leather briefcase. If you want to be taken seriously, consider yourself a professional, and always look the part.

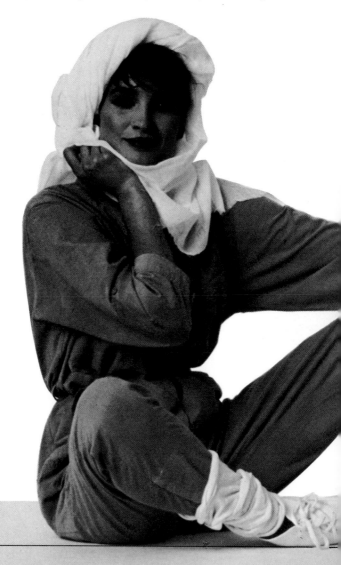

*Defying fashion by wearing clothes you feel right in is preferable to looking like a shop-window dummy. Always remember that your clothes are a projection of character as well as a means of highlighting your best assets.*

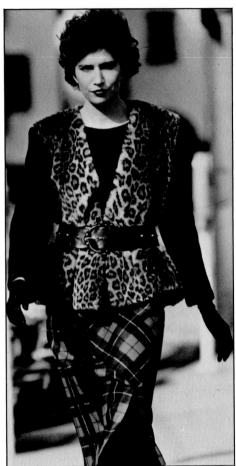

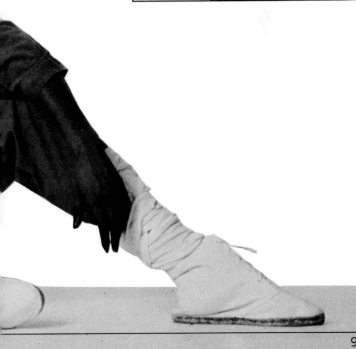

We all have instincts about clothing, and an inner sense of what is right and wrong for ourselves. You know what it feels like to try on clothes that are either too bright, prim, outrageous or bulky. You know how awkward some clothes and accessories can make you feel; conversely, you know how your favorite clothes and accessories instantly inject you with self-assurance. The most efficient way to discover your personal style is to experiment with different looks. Try out new outfits or accessories in front of friends and get their reactions. Never experiment with a new hairstyle, exotic outfit or iridescent earrings on the day of an important interview — you should feel comfortable and confident on such occasions. The idea is to find a style that enhances your looks and complements your personality and to stick with it, refining it with jewelry, belts, scarves, or makeup.

Because style is a very personal thing — less connected with clothes than personality — it is perhaps the only thing you should not attempt to copy. It is no use trying to look like a blonde bombshell if you are dark and demure, or vice versa. It is more important to consider clothes as a projection of character, a means of highlighting your best assets. Defying fashion by wearing clothes you feel like wearing is preferable to looking like a store-window dummy. Remember that the most stylish people appear natural because they have become part of the clothes they wear.

The first step towards cultivating a personal style is to take a critical look at your wardrobe, throwing away the things you feel unhappy in. Then spend an hour or two trying on your favorite clothes and rearranging them. Shorten a dress with a wide belt or wear a sweater back-to-front. If you are feeling adventurous, try wearing a shirt and tie instead of a blouse and a string of pearls. But above all, make sure your clothes feel like you.

## DRESS SENSE: DO'S AND DON'TS

**Do** make colors work for you by selecting shades that complement your shape. Remember that dark colors reduce and light colors enlarge.

**Do** explore less conventional clothes outlets like menswear shops, children's departments, army and navy stores and rummage sales. These are excellent places to discover 'cheap chic'.

**Do** pay more for high-quality coats, jackets and accessories, as they will last for years and add style to cheaper garments.

**Do** take stock of your wardrobe now and then and throw away clothes you have worn out or no longer care for. It is sometimes worth swapping clothes with friends or arranging a temporary exchange, as this is one way to extend your wardrobe.

**Do** develop your own style by wearing clothes you feel happy in and that reflect your personality.

**Do not** spend too much money on basics like skirts and trousers, as they can always be dressed up or down with the right accessories.

**Do not** wear the same colors every year Experiment with color combinations. colour combinations.

**Do not** overload your wardrobe. Choose your clothes carefully for maximum wear and impact.

**Do not** wear clothes you are not comfortable in. It will show.

**Do not** become a slave to fashion. Try and incorporate the latest trends into your own style of dressing, but don't buy something unflattering just because it is in vogue.

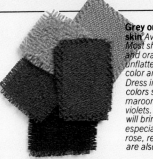

**An astute fashion sense** means realizing that no matter how much you may *like a certain color*, it could be totally wrong for your skin tone. You must also remember that your eyes will usually absorb and *reflect the color of whatever you are wearing. Emphasize the coloring of your complexion, eyes or hair by wearing colors and accessories that enhance your natural looks. The listings below will help you select the right colors for your particular complexion and hair coloring.*

**Red hair and pale skin**
*Avoid strong, striking colors such as purple, red, fuchsia, light green, bright yellow and orange. Stark white is also unadvisable. The best shades are grey and blue, and subdued pastels. Black and beige are always good choices for this coloring.*

**Blonde hair and olive skin**
*Shades such as pale yellow, mustard, lime and off-white emphasize a sallow complexion. Also be careful with pinks, oranges and dark reds. Shades that are right for olive skin include blue, tur-quoise, pale green, grey, charcoal blue and black. Also try bright reds, metallic colours and cocoa brown to make the coordination of your clothing and clothing and coloring truly striking.*

**Blonde hair and fair skin**
*High voltage colors like deep purple, electric blue, shocking pink, fuchsia and orange will overpower your hair and complexion. So will mustard-yellow and brown, bright reds and bright greens. There are, however, a host of shades that look wonderful on fair-skinned blondes, including pale pink, pink-beige, tan, khaki, gold, light grey, white, pale blue, violet, royal blue, navy, lavender, plum and maroon. Green hues such as olive, grass green and forest green are extremely flattering to this color and skin tone and almost any shade of pastel will suit.*

**Grey or silver hair and fair skin** *Avoid wearing pastels. Most shades of yellow, grey and orange will also be unflattering to your hair color and complexion. Dress in classic, dark colors such as black, navy, maroon, deep browns and violets. All shades of blue will bring out your color especially turquoise. Dusty rose, reds, and dark pink are also favorable colors to*

**Brunette and olive skin**
*You will look super-sophisticated in black, charcoal grey, forest green, olive green, khaki green, and off-white. Never wear pastels such as light yellow or bright green; these colors will clash with your complexion. Other colors that will suit you are scarlet, wine red and deep purple.*

**Brunette and fair skin** *You should wear any dark tones that reflect the color of your hair, such as deep reds or chestnut browns. Stay away from beiges and off-whites, as they may make you look paler. Violet, mauve, purple, black, gold, navy, grey, red and pastel colors are the best choices. Also try deep pink, pure white and grey.*

**Light-brown hair and olive skin** *The best range of colors for this combination is dark green, green-blue, grey, grey-blue, navy, black, plum, cherry, red and beige. Intense purples and violets, fuchsia, shocking pink, coral, orange, canary yellow, are all too intense for you and may make your complexion seem unduly olive or sallow.*

**Light-brown hair and fair skin** *Avoid pale greens and yellows, olive green or tan, as they may make your complexion look sallow. Primary colors, and the shades they make when combined, are good choices for you, especially colors like blue-green black, red-rose, pink and off-white. Certain purple shades, like lilac, mauve and grape, also look well on you.*

## Cheap chic

The saying 'It's not what you wear, it's the way that you wear it' must appeal to anyone buying clothes on a tight budget, and the fact is that it is true. From making your own accessories to visiting the children's department in a large store, there are 101 ways to dress cheaply and stylishly. A favourite with many models is army and navy stores where they can buy crisp white painter's overalls, grandad vests, plimsoles and jumpsuits, all of which can be converted into fashionable outfits with the addition of ordinary trousers or a tight belt. For those with a petite figure, children's clothes are not only cheap but often fit better too. 'T' shirts, shorts and even pajamas can be bought at a fraction of the adult price and look just as good as those purchased in the women's department. The menswear department is also perfect for 'cheap chic' finds. A large spacious jacket worn over tight-fitting jeans accentuates feminine curves or hides unsightly bulges.

Rummage sales are still excellent places to discover bargains, particularly the nostalgic variety. Slim pencil skirts and short sixties dresses are usually preferable to their modern counterparts and cost much less. Cheap accessories can be made out of anything from a dyed dishtowel to a dog leash. An unusual necklace can be created in a night by threading strips of suede onto elastdic and separating the various colors with beads. If you lack the patience to make such things, try cutting 'T' shirts into vests and use the remnants as a headband.

*Clothes need not cost you a fortune. With some skill and imagination, you can make something from scratch or adapt an existing garment to a more fashionable style.*

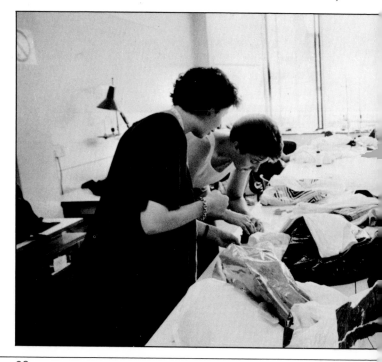

## Natural versus synthetic

Despite the popularity of natural fabrics, most synthetic fibers have just as many advantages as disadvantages. Wool, cotton, silk and linen tend to look and feel better, but these materials are often more expensive and much harder to take care of. However, natural fabrics do allow the skin to breathe and are therefore better for underwear and sporting gear. By comparison, synthetic fibers are cheaper and stand up to the wear and tear, making them a perfect choice for packing into a suitcase.

## The sophisticated look

Fashion sense means knowing how to combine different elements successfully, being able to see and judge the overall effect of your clothing and accessories, and, finally, realizing when your clothes and accessories clash or are simply inappropriate for certain situations. The most practical way to develop your personal fashion sense is to study the top women's fashion magazines and criticize their pictures with an objective eye. Familiarize yourself with the work of the top fashion designers and photographers and get an idea of the current fashion. Analyze the styles, fabrics and colors. Try to imagine what outfits would look well on you, and which ones would be unsuitable. Consider yourself fortunate if you know how to sew, because you can buy commercial patterns copied from designer clothes. You can create perfectly tailored outfits or separates in the current fashion for a more economical price than store-bought clothing.

Use your instincts when shopping for clothes and accessories, but also try to see yourself as others see you. Wear anything you want to in your leisure time — just remember that you must choose a work wardrobe that is suited to your particular office environment.

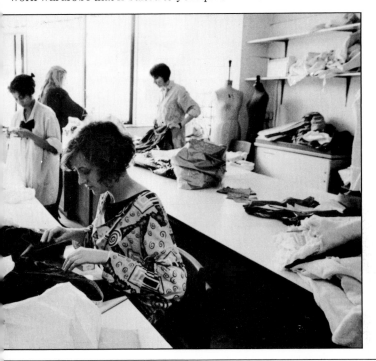

We all have instincts about clothes — a sense of what is right and wrong for ourselves. So, to discover your personal style, experiment with different looks, color combinations, shapes and types of fabric. The sketches on these pages illustrate how you can use swatches of fabric, buttons and other materials to design an outfit.

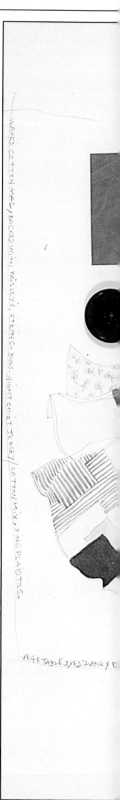

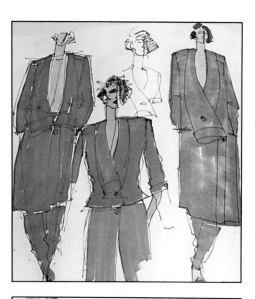

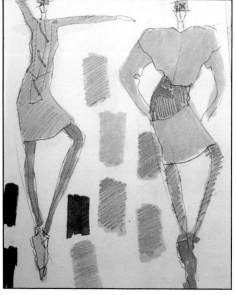

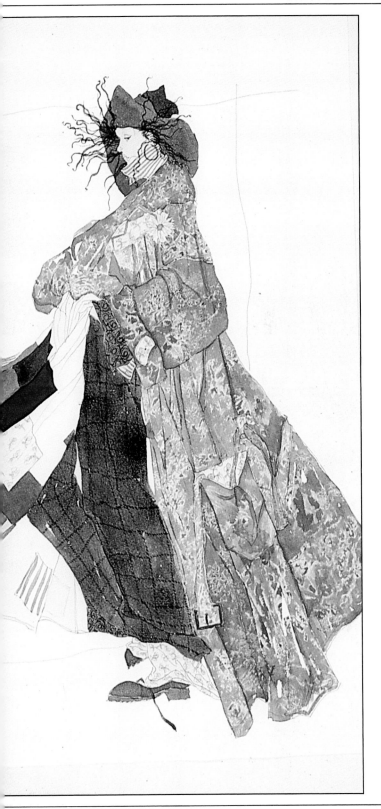

## Complementing your figure

Not surprisingly, the shape of your body will determine what styles and fabrics you can wear. The following guidelines should help you in selecting figure-flattering clothes.

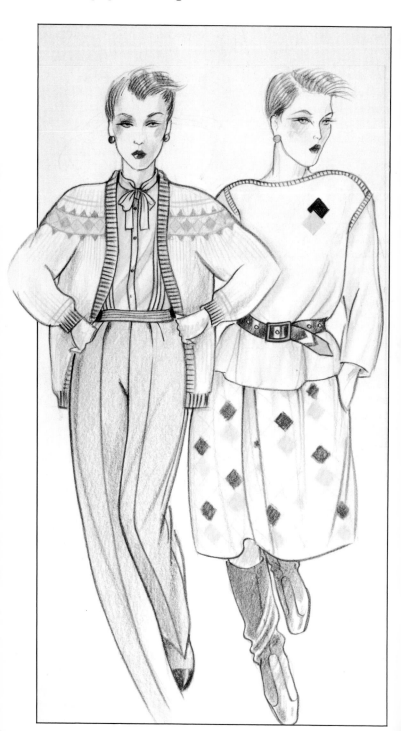

# Hips

Hip measurements differ greatly from woman to woman. This can be a source of great frustration, and women who buy their clothes in department stores often complain that standard sizings do not correspond to their measurements. The truth of this situation is borne out by a recent survey, which discovered that 50 per cent of women who buy their clothes in stores and boutiques — or sew them from patterns — have to alter them to make them fit. If your hips are wide and well-padded, you must reconcile yourself to the fact that you will never look petite. Do not wear anything with a tight waist, any clinging fabrics, or brightly patterned trousers, skirts and dresses. Heavily textured fabrics, knitted garments, and pleated skirts are also best avoided. Instead, wear gored skirts, tailored trousers in dark colors, and boxy jackets. Dark-colored jumpsuits will make your hips look slimmer, but be sure to wear matching shoes or boots with them to give an unbroken line of color. Wearing earrings, or trying a colorful scarf around your neck, will help distract the eye from the hip area. You can also try wearing hats that match the colors of your sweaters or blouses.

Accentuating slim hips is very easy to carry off, as there are many outfits you can wear to make your figure look shapely. Form-fitting designer jeans or plain blue jeans look very flattering worn with a blouse tucked in at the waist and a wide leather belt. Heavy, textured fabrics, like hard-woven wools or corduroys, are the best materials for trousers and skirts, and knitted skirts and dresses in striped patterns and vibrant colors also work well. Simultaneously comfortable, functional and attractive, pastel or bright-colored jumpsuits are excellent clothing choices for women with slim hips. Wear them with woven sashes or leather belts at the waist. In the past few years, the fashion pendulum has swung back to the mini-length skirt and dress styles of the swinging '60s. If your slim hips and shapely legs look good in short skirt lengths, then wear a dress or skirt above the knee.

# Legs

If you have short legs, do not wear skirts and dresses with pleats, ruffles, flounces or any other features that will highlight your leg area. The best way to de-emphasize this characteristic is by dressing in matching dark-colored separates with matching shoes. This unbroken line of color will give a slimming and length-ening illusion to your figure. Always be sure to match the color of your hose with your skirts and shoes. Forget about patterned or light-colored hose — black or navy sheer hosiery will look best on your legs. When selecting shoes and boots, always look for thin-heeled footwear that will add height to your figure. Short legs and heavy legs are not flattered by ankle-straps or sling-back shoe styles. Chunky-heeled shoes like clogs are especially uncomplimentary, and never wear boots that are calf-length, or knee-high boots that hug your calf. If your ankles are thick, look for fine, soft leather boots that fit loosely around the ankles. In general, you want to make your feet and legs as inconspicuous as possible, so stick with dark tones and suedes whenever possible.

If your legs are very thin, you can enhance their shape and size by wearing light-colored hose — white and bone, lilac and yellow, or patterned. With the myriad of styles available in stores and boutiques, you can find anything from white printed with Matisse-like flowers to orange and black tiger-stripe designs. There are also more conservative styles, such as seamed or clocked hose (clocking is a term for a tiny, embroidered design on the sides of the legs or at the ankles). These hosiery styles work well for office or evening wear, but stick with light-to-medium shades.

## How to conceal a large stomach

There are a few tried and tested ground rules to follow if you have this common figure problem. The first is to avoid wearing anything that terminates at your waistline, such as boxy jackets, vests, blouses or wide sashes and belts. Avoid tight-fitting clothes and thick, textured fabrics that tend to emphasize the contours of your body. Never wear dirndls, as these will draw attention to your stomach. Instead, try wearing tailored, A-line dresses that stop just below the knee. Empire waistlines are also flattering to this shape, and tunics with a narrow belt of matching fabric over skirts or pants will make your waist look slimmer. Solid, dark colors are best and remember that prints and patterns tend to make your body look larger, so keep your style simple and classic. You may also want to wear figure-flattering lingerie such as girdles or 'all-in-ones', as these can give the illusion of a flatter stomach. Girdles hold in the stomach and buttocks, but a one-piece suit consisting of a bra, an elasticized stomach panel, and panties are better. The prime advantage of an all-in-one is that it gives your body a unified line under your clothes, while a girdle stops at your waist and will be visible through many lightweight fabrics. Another way to divert attention from your stomach is to wear jackets, blouses or dresses that have built-in shoulder pads. Shoulder pads broaden the shoulder line, thereby creating the illusion of a more evenly proportioned body.

## Making the most of a small bust

If you are a dancer or a model a small bust is an asset, as clothing will drape quite easily and elegantly on your body. With small breasts you also have unlimited clothing options. You can wear vests, blouses and sweaters without a bra. If you want to make a small bust look fuller, try wearing a padded bra or several layers of clothing in coordinated patterns or shades.

## How to make a large bust look smaller

There are several tactics you can adopt to make a large bust less obvious. If you want to look smaller all the time, then only wear dark-coloured blouses, sweaters and jackets. Do not wear knitted vests or any garment that is tight-fitting on top. Never wear bows around your collar or double-breasted styles. Give away anything in your closet that has a large pattern or boisterous color scheme and avoid wearing shiny fabrics or billowing, peasant blouses. Go for outfits with rounded or 'V' necklines and avoid turtlenecks and square necklines. Experiment with earrings to find styles that suit you, as attractive earrings will help to draw attention away from your bustline.

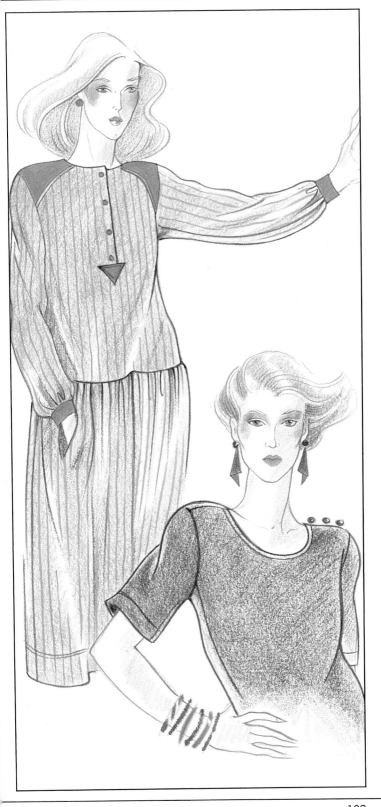

# THE RIGHT ATTITUDE

In the final analysis, your attitude will always be more valuable than your looks, for a positive attitude is what draws (and keeps) people close to you. One of the most telling indicators of attitude is the tempo and volume of the voice. Most people have very little idea of what their voice really sounds like because it is distorted when it resonates in the head. Make a tape recording of your voice and listen carefully; identify its characteristics. Is the tone surprisingly nasal? Is your diction well-articulated, or do you tend to mumble your speech? Are you a hurried or a slow talker? Some people have a permanently deadpan pitch to their voice, implying, perhaps wrongly, that they are bored or uninterested. Once you become aware of what your voice sounds like, you can start exercising control over its volume, articulation, pitch and speed. Most people prefer to hear low-pitched, slow voices, but if yours is high, simply try to speak as clearly and naturally as possible.

Another factor that contributes to a positive attitude is the ability to listen attentively and choose questions carefully. The fact is, you can talk to anybody about practically anything if you make a conscious effort to receive and absorb their message.

Finally, make sure that you go into every situation with an open, yet critical mind. This will enable you to get the most out of your experience. Prejudging people, ideas, customs or works of art before you truly comprehend them is a negative habit that we all share. This character trait can lose you potential friends, jobs, knowledge and pleasure. Don't fall prey to it, but if you recognize it in yourself, then examine what might cause you to be so critical or harsh. The chances are that something about the person or idea in question is vaguely threatening to you. It's alright to be insecure, but confront and recognize your insecurity as such. Instead of trying to change your normal speech pattern or tense your facial muscles into a grinning, frozen mask, simply admit to yourself when you're under pressure and try to be as natural as possible. Personnel officers and other professionals expect you to be slightly nervous in an interview or important meeting. To diffuse your nervousness, realize that other people have faced far more gruelling circumstances and handled them with ease. Ernest Hemingway's classic definition, 'Courage is grace under pressure,' should put the challenges you face into their proper perspective.

*Even if you are blessed with stunning good looks, you still won't get far as a model unless you have confidence. Both Jane Fonda (right) and Jerry Hall (far right) possess a high degree of self-assurance and vitality.*

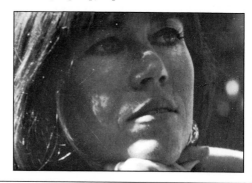

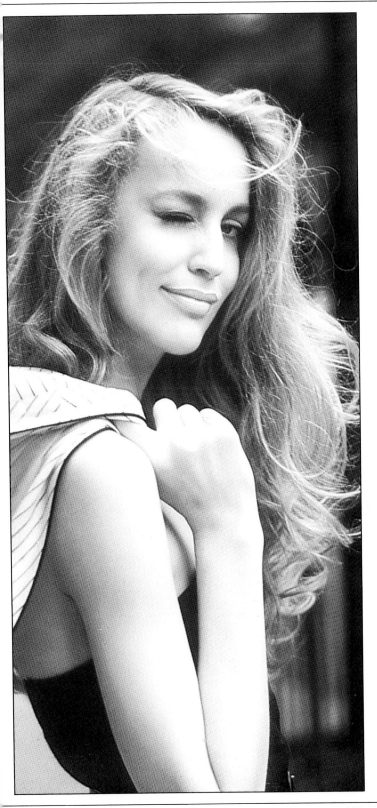

# ACCESSORIES

The kind of accessories you wear should be determined by your bone structure and build. If you have a large frame you can wear medium to large scarves and belts. You can also wear jewellery such as multiple gold chains, charms and pearls to great effect. What you should avoid, however, are tiny rings, pins and thin bangle bracelets. A finer-boned woman will want to limit herself to smaller-scale accessories. Delicate scarves, light jewelry, functional but streamlined handbags — these all harmonize well with fine features. This is not to say that you can't wear a large, silver belt buckle or a huge leather saddlebag purse, if you are petite. The important thing

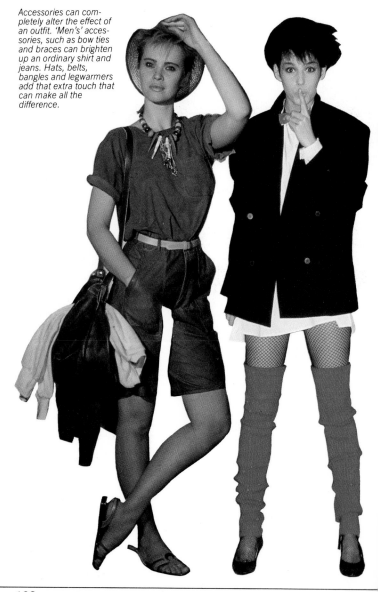

Accessories can completely alter the effect of an outfit. 'Men's' accessories, such as bow ties and braces can brighten up an ordinary shirt and jeans. Hats, belts, bangles and legwarmers add that extra touch that can make all the difference.

to remember is balance. Do not wear several large items together, or you will look weighed down by your accessories.

The great benefit of jewelry and scarves, hosiery and belts, bags, hats and gloves is that they can be used not only to harmonize with your features and clothing, but they can also show off the texture of your clothes or hair. A patterned silk scarf, for instance, can draw attention to the delicate knit of your alpaca sweater, while a classic Scottish tweed jacket will look dashing with a string of pearls and a red wool muffler. Polished wooden beads or glazed ceramic ones will emphasize heavy winter-textured clothes and thick, curly hair. Belts can also be used to contrast with the material of your sweaters, blouses, skirts or trousers. Don't be afraid to try new combinations of accessories; they can help stretch a basic wardrobe a long way.

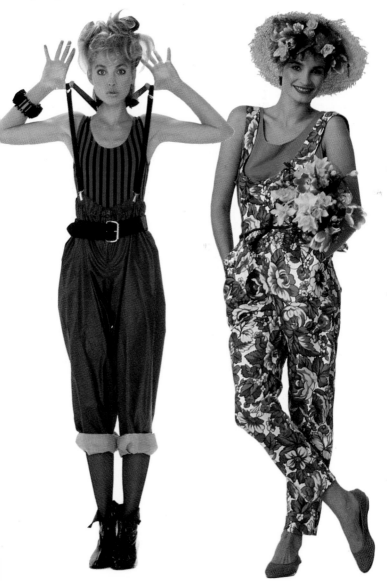

# 4
# THE MODELING WORLD

## FIELDS OF MODELING

## A MODEL'S DAY

## STAYING IN SHAPE

## THE PORTFOLIO

## PHOTO SESSIONS

## SHOOTING ON LOCATION

## MODELLING AGENCIES

*T*here are many factors to take into consideration before you embark on a modelling career and it is therefore important to know all about the various fields before you sign with an agency and start competing with other models for assignments. A model has a relatively brief career, but the financial rewards can be considerable. With a strong personality, a professional attitude and a photogenic appearance you have the right basic ingredients for success.

# FIELDS OF MODELING

Models are generally divided into two market types: *fashion* and *commercial*. That is to say, you have the looks and style for certain types of photographic and/or show modeling, or your looks and talent are most appropriate for print and television advertising. The classic, female, fashion type is considered to be from 5ft 7in to 5ft 11in, with well-defined bone structure, wide-set eyes, long legs, and a perfectly proportioned dress size of 10 or 12. Commercial-looking models can range from sporty, long-haired blondes to conservatively attractive career women. Less publicized modeling types include child models and feature models. Feature modeling refers to the modeling of legs, hands, hair, feet and individual facial features. Both child and feature models are consistently in demand by magazines, catalogs, print and television advertisers, and can earn salaries equivalent to those of the top fashion models of the moment. There are also two types of modeling that do not fall into standard categories — these are lingerie and nude modelling.

There are many models in the business who possess the requisite qualities for working in several areas. A typical week's bookings for a busy model in a major city might include: two fashion shows, three magazine photo sessions and a television commercial for lingerie that calls for leg modeling only. There also happen to be a good number of child models who regularly do magazine (also called editorial) and catalogue work, as well as occasional advertising shoots. Child models who have strong performing skills as well as supportive parents are in an excellent position to pursue a career in television commercials.

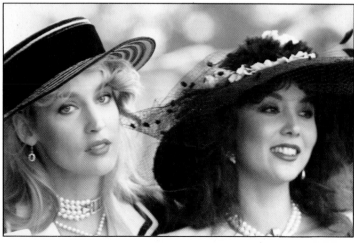

*Jerry Hall (above left) and Marie Helvin (above and right) are both top photographic and show models. Tall and slim, they have cover-girl qualities: high cheekbones, full sensual mouths and wide eyes.*

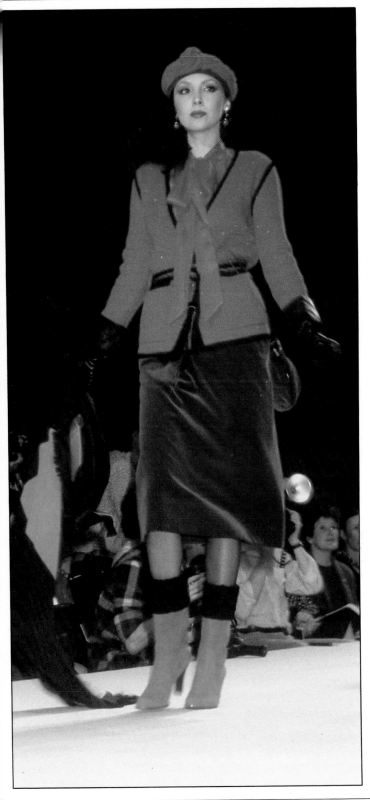

## Editorial photographic modeling

'Fashion editors are interested in extremely tall, thin models with a striking appearance. Strong features like high cheekbones, a full, sensual mouth and wide eyes — these are cover-girl qualities,' says Anne Soorikian, a beauty editor on *McCall's* magazine. 'A model for editorial print fashion spreads has to have a lean, well-toned body that looks terrific in bathing suits, evening clothes, you name it...Because of the contemporary physical fitness trend, the athletic beauty of models like Christie Brinkley and Patti Hansen is replacing the super-thin looking model in popularity. Women who have exotic faces can also expect to achieve success in photographic modeling. This is because racially and ethnically-mixed looks are perennially sought after by the top fashion magazines, although they are largely ignored by other sectors of the industry.'

Like Anne Soorikian, Susan Shilling has been working with fashion publications for several years. Susan is the studio manager for the internationally famous fashion photographer Francesco Scavullo. Acclaimed for his cover photography, fashion spreads and portraiture for magazines such as *Cosmopolitan, Harper's Bazaar* and Italian *Vogue*, Scavullo photographs top models and celebrities for a wide variety of editorial and advertising shots. As studio manager, Susan works in conjunction with Scavullo, his clients and modeling agencies, to select the appropriate models for each session. She offers the following tips on what qualities can help a photographic model's career:

● Nine times out of ten, clients prefer models with adaptable hairstyles. For maximum versatility, wear your hair in a shoulder-length blunt cut. Never change the style or color of your hair without first consulting your agency.

● Treat the clothes and accessories that you are modeling with the utmost consideration. Always put your clothes on *after* you have applied your makeup, for instance. Wear an anti-perspirant so that you do not stain your clothes. In many cases, the outfits worn by models are one-of-a-kind designer's samples. As such, they must be returned to the client's factory or showroom in good condition so that they can be copied. The care that you take in handling your client's clothing can help you to build up a good reputation in the business.

● Cultivate your ability to cooperate with and take directions from clients and photographers. Part of a photographic model's job involves understanding the client's marketing approach, and expressing that approach through a variety of poses and nuances. 'A truly professional model has more than one face, more than one look.'

Susan goes on to explain: 'A good model knows how to wear and display clothes made from different fabrics. For example, she will instinctively know how to move in a material such as silk in order to show it to its best advantage. She will also feel good in the clothes she is wearing because she has a familiarity with her body that is based on a combination of experience and self-awareness... Another example of skilled modeling is someone who can wear layers and layers of clothing with a vital energy and individuality and who knows how to work with the different parts of the outfit so that she is more than just a human hanger. A good model will go to each booking and ask herself "What is the purpose of this session? What image does the client want to create?" She knows that the point of the shoot is to project a particular fashion look or product; she never thinks of how to project herself'.

## Catalog modeling

Models with wholesome, attractive, but 'undramatic' looks tend to get the most work in this field. Even-featured looks are the norm. Blondes and brown-haired models are more in demand than dark-haired, sultry types. It is not uncommon for models who are nearing the end of their print careers to make the transition to catalog modeling, as age requirements are far less stringent. Although many models consider catalog work less glamorous and interesting than editorial print work, it can be a far more lucrative and secure field of modeling.

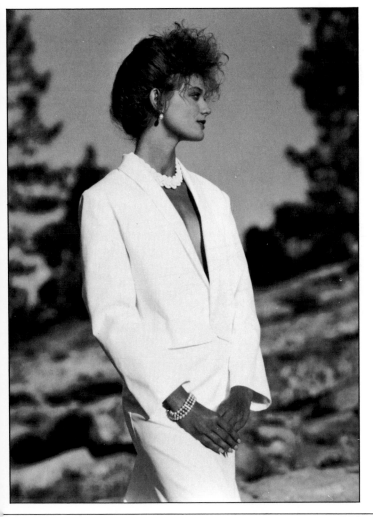

## Shows and collection modeling

A 'live' model, or *mannequin*, does not need to have the beautiful, photogenic features of the average photographic model. Because fashion shows are a type of performance, a mannequin must radiate the essence of the clothes she wears through her gestures, through her walk, through her persona. A mannequin is an integral element of a designer or clothing company's fashion collection. She will be judged not so much for her looks as for her style.

Mannequins play a major role in the success (and failure) of fashion collections. By wearing the clothing in an expressive and spirited way, they stimulate interest in the clothes, and they

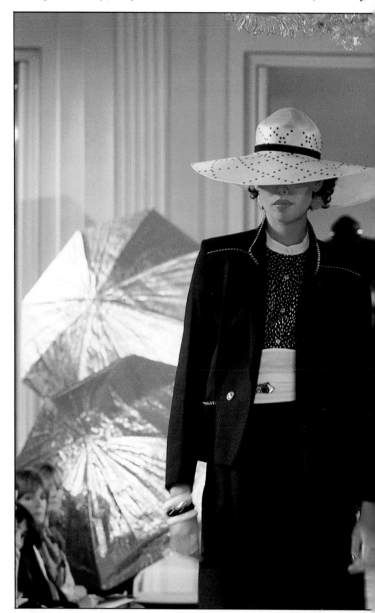

are largely responsible for the sales orders that come in after the show from department stores and private buyers. 'They alone give life to my dresses,' said the great French couturier, Christian Dior — 'I cannot think of one without the other.' Mannequins also influence the taste and decisions of the powerful fashion press, who report on and feature each season's new clothes and accessories for their readers. An enthusiastic review of a collection can boost a designer's status (and profits) in the space of a few weeks. A good mannequin knows this, and does everything she can to interpret her designer's fashions in a fresh and exciting display as she models in a showroom or glides down the catwalk at a fashion show.

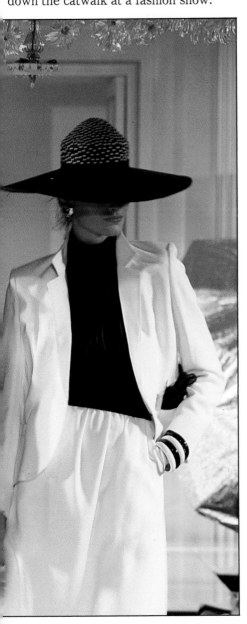

*Mannequins or 'live' models are judged not so much for their looks as for their style. They can make or break a fashion collection.*

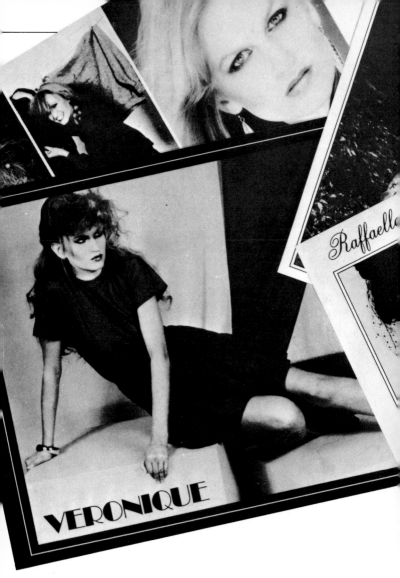

VERONIQUE

Raffaell

## Haute couture modeling

*Haute couture* is French for 'high fashion' and refers to the clothes that are custom-made for private clients by a specific designer or 'couturier'. Certain *haute couture* designers, such as Coco Chanel, Yves Saint Laurent and Bill Blass, have been setting the standards for women's fashion for decades, and to be a mannequin for their shows can be a marvelously glamorous experience. It should be noted that show modeling pays much less than photographic modeling, but, if a designer likes the way you move, you will probably be asked to model repeatedly for future shows. It is not unusual for *couture* models to continue modeling well into their thirties.

Holly Henley, formerly an *haute couture* mannequin for Paris-based designers, including Emmanuel Ungaro and Pierre Cardin, got her start in the business by showing up (uninvited) at designers' salons as they were nearing the autumn collection season: 'There is always a need for models around the autumn

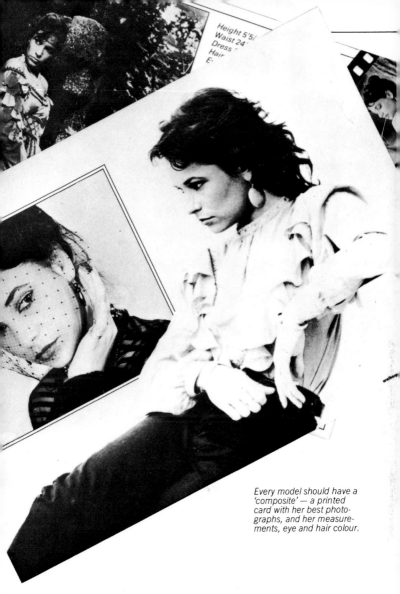

Every model should have a 'composite' — a printed card with her best photographs, and her measurements, eye and hair colour.

and spring collection times, and, since I knew how to walk, they hired me on the spot. I hadn't had much experience, but the Europeans are not as professionally oriented as they are in New York. European fashion is more artistic than commercial; the attitude is more spontaneous and creative. Models in Europe will earn substantially less than American show or photographic models, but the experience makes it worthwhile. You can develop your style, do some impressive work, and immerse yourself in fashion before going elsewhere in search of an agency and better-paid jobs.'

As a rule, *haute couture* mannequins are supplied to designers by modeling agencies. If you want to be a show model, the best way to pursue this is by making an appointment with an agency. They will ask you to walk for them and then they will decide if they can find you work. They will not be interested in hiring you unless your height and dress size are within the required range.

## Modeling for commercials

There are two ways to pursue a career in this field of modeling. You can either try for representation by a reputable theatrical agency, or you can try affiliating yourself with a major modeling agency. The top modeling agencies all have 'talent' divisions that handle bookings for television commercial work. If you are already a photographic or advertising model, then the odds are good that you will eventually land some parts in commercials. Television advertisers tend to hire models and actors who range from wholesome, healthy types to more sophisticated (but not too exotic) fashion models. The performing skills that they all must have are enthusiasm, naturalness and sincerity. Good teeth, attractive hair and a pleasant, unaccented speaking voice are absolute musts for aspiring commercial models. If your voice is thin and high, however, you can be dubbed over by a more suitable voice. You stand to make much more money if you have a speaking part in a commercial, so take diction or voice lessons to increase your commercial potential.

To make it in commercial and advertising modeling, you need not have the beautiful attributes of a high-fashion photographic model. You are not expected to fulfil the specific height, weight or size requirements that govern so many areas of modeling. Although it is encouraging that more and more commercial and print advertisers are hiring models of Black and Asian extraction, the people chosen usually possess rather 'Westernized' features, such as narrow, even noses, thin lips and wide-set eyes. But according to Shelly Hamilton, a New York television commercial casting director, 'The racial bias is continuing to lessen as big corporations begin to realize that for certain products, a more compelling, ethnic face can sell the product to a wider audience than any Caucasian ones can.'

There is room for as many types of models in advertising print modeling as there are products on the market. If your agency thinks that you have potential for advertising modeling, then you are fortunate. Not only can it be highly paid, but you will have the satisfaction of seeing your face in newspapers, magazines, and maybe on billboards. The most successful models in this field are tall, brown-haired or blonde types who can sell a product and look appealing at the same time. This is harder than it sounds, because many models find that their looks are too exotic, too sensual or too stunning. Advertisers are primarily interested in finding models to whom a mass consumer audience can relate.

*Successful advertising models are those who can sell a product and look appealing at the same time. If, like this model (right) you are advertising tights, then obviously you would be required to have long, shapely legs as well.*

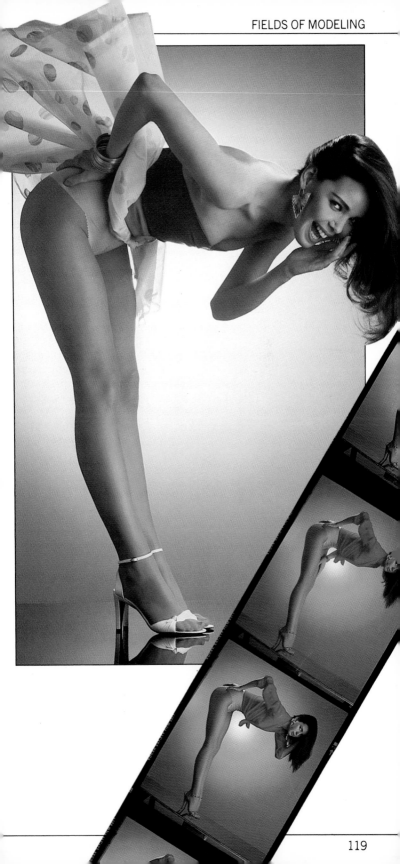

Small-boned women with long, slender, shapely legs and delicate ankles are usually selected as leg models. It can be a very tiring form of modeling as it often involves long photo sessions with hours of standing, sometimes in high heels.

If you are fortunate enough to have shiny, luxurious hair, you may find an opening in advertising hair-products.

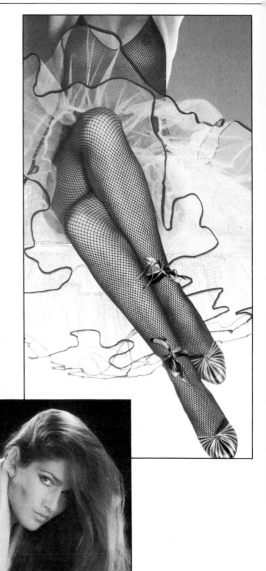

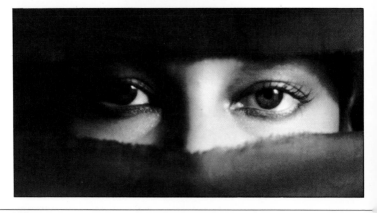

## Feature modeling

Print advertisers frequently work with models in this category. For example, toothpaste advertisements need close-ups of the mouth; packagers of hosiery need legs; jewellery and cosmetics companies often use hand models to advertise their products. Department store advertisements and catalogues use a great number of feature models, and there is also a certain amount of editorial print work for feature models. How do you know if you can do this kind of modeling? The answer is that you must have absolutely flawless hands, legs, eyes or whatever feature is required, and a modeling agency is the best judge of this. It is generally agreed that the basic qualities required of hand models are: long, slender fingers, tapered fingertips, narrow palms and immaculately manicured nails. Hand modeling can be quite tiring — the positions that you have to hold can cramp your hands halfway through the session, and if you can't keep that jar of cold cream steady, the photographer will not get the pictures that he or she needs.

With regard to leg models, agencies and clients usually hire tall, small-boned women with long, shapely slender legs and delicate ankles. Show models often do leg modeling as well, since the posing techniques are somewhat similar. Models agree, however, that leg modeling is exceedingly strenuous because it requires many long hours of standing and a photo session can be doubly uncomfortable if the model is given high heels to wear. A leg model could benefit immensely from a disciplined exercise regime — whether it is dance classes, jogging, or working out with weights. 'You'll need muscular strength and good circulation for this kind of physical work,'advises Beth Rubino, an American photographic and television model who is also a top New York bodybuilder.

If you are fortunate enough to have almond-shaped eyes, then you may have what it takes to do eye modeling. Other eye shapes, of course, are used by advertisers and editorial art directors, but almond eyes seem to be a perennial favorite of cosmetics advertisers and beauty magazines. Other characteristics considered outstanding in this field are purple, light green and bright blue eyes; thick, upswept eyebrows, long eyelashes and slanted eyes.

Mouth models are expected to have perfectly shaped, white teeth. The lip shape can vary from thin and wide to full and pouty. As long as the proportions between the teeth, lips and upper lip are pleasingly even, then a model with bright white teeth is well endowed for mouth modeling. Needless to say, if you hope to do any type of facial modeling, expert makeup skills are required.

## Lingerie and nude modeling

Women who model bras, panties, girdles or slips can expect to earn two to three times more than their regular hourly agency rate. The drawback of this type of work is that one tends to get 'typecast' as a lingerie model. Certain advertising and editorial art directors may be unwilling to use models who have appeared, or are currently appearing, in national or regional lingerie advertisements, commercials or catalogues. If your agency thinks you have potential for this kind of work, however, and you can accept the fact that this may preclude you from being a success in other fields of modeling, then perhaps you should do a few lingerie bookings. At the very least, you will be well paid for them, and if you don't like the photographs, leave them out of your professional portfolio.

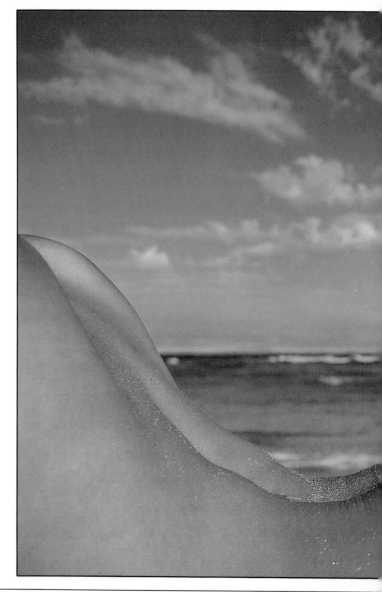

Nude modeling for editorial and advertising purposes fetches the highest hourly and daily rates in the business. Many models who do this type of work often exclude it from their portfolios, especially if their faces are visible in the photographs. Nude modeling is not considered to be a particularly useful stepping stone to other areas of the industry. It could harm your chances of ever doing high fashion photographic work, television commercials or show modeling. But, if you want to do feature modeling or lingerie work, some artistic and tasteful nude shots in your portfolio may help you to get some prestigious or lucrative bookings.

*Nude modeling is well paid but unless tastefully undertaken, not necessarily helpful to a model's career.*

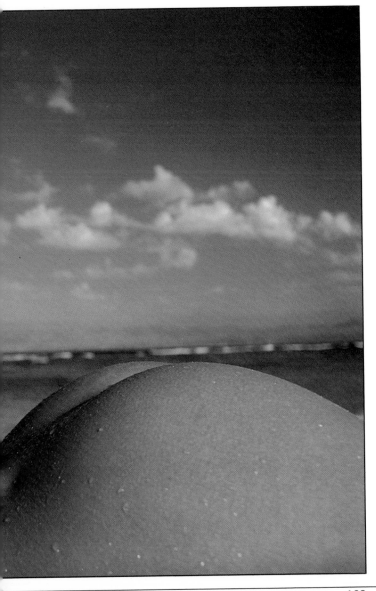

# A MODEL'S DAY

A professional model's typical working day often demands that she rise between 6 and 7am for an early morning photo session, and it is quite possible that she could work without stopping until 10 or 11pm, if she has an especially time-consuming booking, such as a television commercial. If this seems like an exhausting schedule to you, then consider what her unbooked days can be like: she may have a full day of appointments with photo studio managers, advertising agencies and magazine fashion editors that have been arranged by her agency. Sometimes these appointments will be interviews for a specific booking in the near future, but more often these brief meetings serve the purpose of promoting an agency's newer models to potential clients. It stands to reason that clients will prefer to hire models whom they know — and like — to ones they have only seen in agency brochures.

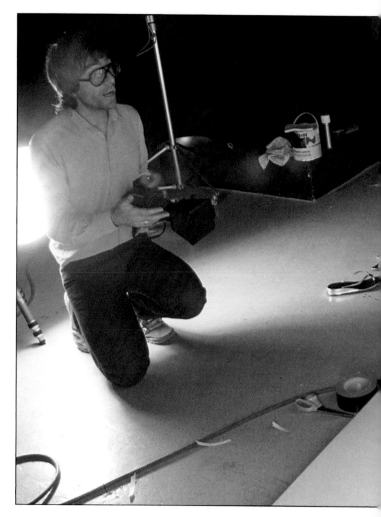

When you meet a client, be both friendly and professional in manner. Show the client your portfolio or book and let him or her peruse it at leisure. Do not comment on your photographs; wait for him or her to ask questions. You will favorably impress prospective clients by being composed, cheerful and straight-forward, because this is undoubtedly the personality type that they will want to work with.

A model's constructive use of her unbooked time can pay off in terms of good rapport with clients or, even better, it may actually net her bookings for one or more shoots. Another way that a model can make her unbooked time work for her is by doing test shots and updating her book with new photographs. A modeling agency can be a great help in suggesting specific kinds of photographs that will enhance her portfolio; it can also arrange sessions with fashion photographers who are interested in testing with new models. Other essential personnel needed for a shoot, such as make-up artists and hair stylists, are usually willing to contribute their services to a model's test shoot in exchange for a print that they can use in their books.

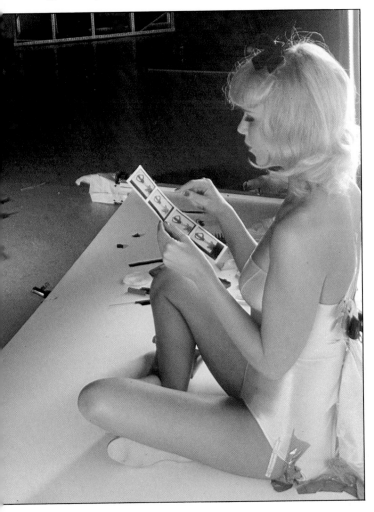

# STAYING IN SHAPE

Once you start getting your first bookings, you will doubtless find that your free time is more scarce. Do not let your work schedule get so hectic that you skip meals or abandon your exercise program. If you are negligent about nutrition and exercise, your looks and health will slide into a visible decline, and, although you may think that you get enough exercise during your workdays, your body still needs programed exercise for optimum health and strength.

Lyne Pedola, a top model with one of New York's most prestigious agencies, The Fords, says this: 'My system is very sensitive, so I do everything I can to stay healthy.' Booked almost constantly, Lyne's schedule demands that she be in perfect shape from head to toe every day of the year. 'You can't afford *not* to take care of yourself in this business, because it could mean having to cancel some of your bookings…Although I know of some models who have terrible eating habits and never exercise, I don't understand how they have the strength to keep on working.' Lyne has been modeling non-stop for seven years, and her abundant engery, sparkling eyes and glowing skin prove that a woman can have a strenuous career and also be supremely healthy and well-groomed. All it takes is planning, and a commitment to a healthy lifestyle.

Although there is a direct link between Lyne's personal care system and her continued success as a model, there is another fundamental reason for her top professional status: her positive, flexible personality. During a fast-paced photo session for a famous department store's spring catalogue, Lyne responded to multiple directions from the clients and photographer with the sureness and calm concentration of an expert. When she tried on a skirt that she was to model and discovered it was four sizes too large, Lyne immediately enlisted the stylist's help for some quick adjustments. In a crowded and tightly-scheduled photo session, an unflappable model can be the salvation of a harried photographer and everyone else involved with the shoot.

*For optimum health and strength, your body needs programmed exercises. So no matter how hectic your work schedule, make sure you eat regularly and work out every day.*

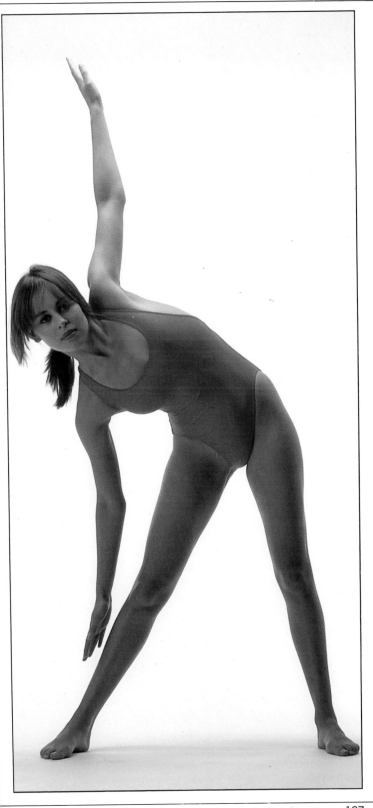

# THE PORTFOLIO

Modeling agencies and their clients share similar goals, but their major goal is finding and working with models who photograph beautifully. Of course a model needs to look attractive, but, above all, her face and body must photograph well from different angles — in black and white *and* color. This is why it is essential for you to assemble a portfolio of 8 x 10in (20 x 24cm) black and white prints, and 12 to 20 good color slides. Your portfolio, or book, as it is called in the profession, should contain three types of 8 x 10in (20 x 24cm) shots and slides: a full-length body shot, a full-face profile and a full-face front. Each of the poses should show a different facial expression and makeup look. Keep the shots simple in composition, standing in front of a wall or seamless studio backdrop. Never use props in these pictures, because the results you want to achieve are sharp, high-contrast photos in which attention is focused on you. Stick with conventional angles and lighting for best results. Before you can do any of this, however, it is necessary first to find a photographer whose work seems to indicate that he or she can take the kind of test shots (portfolio shots) that you need.

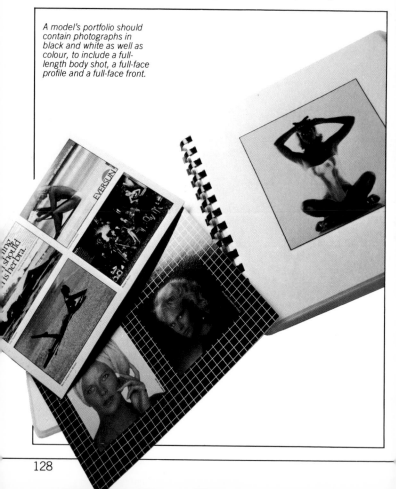

*A model's portfolio should contain photographs in black and white as well as colour, to include a full-length body shot, a full-face profile and a full-face front.*

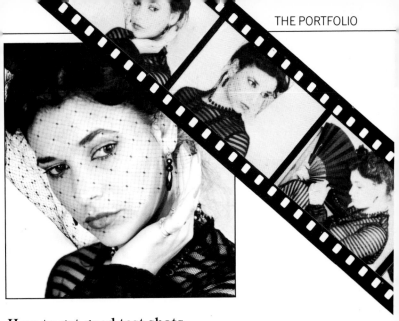

## How to get good test shots

What you are looking for when you are starting out on a modeling career is someone who is just as eager to photograph you as you are willing to be photographed — in short, someone who is interested in test-shooting with new models. Do not offer full payment to the photographer, as you will need several 8 x 10in (20 x 24cm) prints as well as colour slides. What you should do is indicate to the photographer that you will cover the film costs and processing if necessary. There are several ways you can find someone to work with you. If you are at school or college for instance, you may find student photographers who would jump at the chance to do your portfolio shots. Of course, if you have a friend or a relative who is a fairly accomplished photographer, then you could also shoot with them. Remember, you are likely to feel more comfortable being photographed by people you already know. Always meet the photographer and review his or her work before you decide to do a photo session. Make sure that you understand each other regarding the terms of payment and how many contact sheets, slides and prints you will receive after the shoot.

If you live in a major city, you will have no difficulty in finding photographers who specialize in this kind of work. (Some of these photographers will charge a fee, but you will get some highly professional photographs in exchange.) Scan the entertainment industry's weekly newspapers for photographers' advertisements. Another place to find bona fide photographers is in a directory containing information about photographers, advertising, modeling and talent agencies, and the different areas of print and television media. Remember, it is standard practice in this industry to test free of charge.

When you finally find yourself a photographer's studio for test shots, you should be prepared to get the most from this opportunity. Study these guidelines for choosing appropriate clothing, hair styles, make-up and expressions beforehand, and you will have some idea what you are doing.

## Full-length body shots

Wear a simply tailored, short-sleeved or sleeveless dress that shows your legs and arms to good advantage. Do not wear anything excessively tight or loose — go for something classically styled. Your dress should be in either a subdued pattern or a solid color. Do not wear any jewelry except for delicate earrings, such as small hoops or gemstone studs. Stand with your back to the wall, or a seamless backdrop, and let your arms hang in a relaxed manner at your sides. Be as fluid in your movements as possible. Do not be afraid to ask the photographer for direction. Always look directly into the camera and smile. In this kind of shot, you should wear the hairstyle that harmonizes best with the style of your dress, since the goal of this picture is to show off your figure first, and your face second. Start with subtle make-up for this shot, saving your technical wizardry for your head shots.

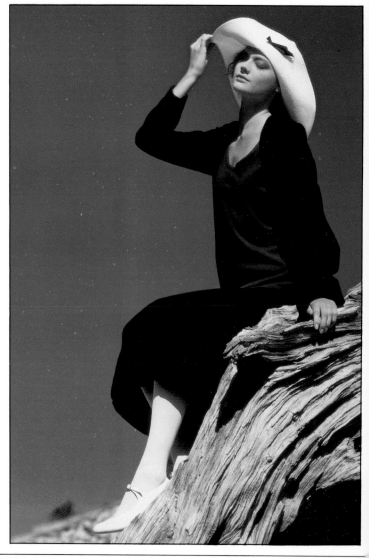

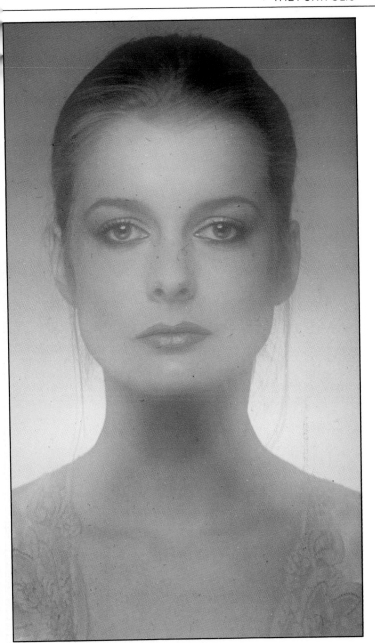

## Full-face front

Wear your hair styled away from your face so your bone structure will be fully appreciated. Wear a blouse with a rounded neckline and do not wear jewelry around your neck. Small earrings are fine if you want to wear them, however. Look directly into the camera and smile, showing your teeth. Try smiling with your mouth closed too, and try to make your eyes expressive in different ways. Shoot against a light-colored background, and experiment with the intensity of your make-up when switching from black and white to color film.

## Full-face profile

Wear your hair pulled back for maximum dramatic effect. Before you start shooting, first decide with the photographer which is your better side. Move your head slightly up and back while the photographer works, and try a three-quarter face position every other shot. Always keep your eyes wide open as you are posing, but do not exaggerate them. Again, maintain a dialogue with the photographer about which moves you should try next. Use contour makeup and eyeshadow to emphasize your features, varying their intensity as you go along. Wear a simple blouse and earrings for this set of shots.

You must be sure that the photographer shoots each of your poses in both black and white and color. Although agencies are primarily interested in seeing black and white test shots, you may want to spend the extra money and make prints from successful color slides for your book. After your shots are processed and you are presented with the contact sheets, take the time to review them with a critical eye. Are these photographs appropriate for your book? You will need six good, high-contrast photographs with different expressions to show how photogenic you are. If you are less than pleased with your shots, then you should definitely try testing again. Your book must be perfect, and it is better to go through testing a few times rather than use photographs that are not quite right.

When you get some pictures that you are proud of, have about thirty 8 x 10in (20 x 25.5cm) black and white prints made up of the very best shot. Type your name, address and phone number on adhesive labels and stick these on the back of each photograph. A creative idea to try (if you can afford the extra

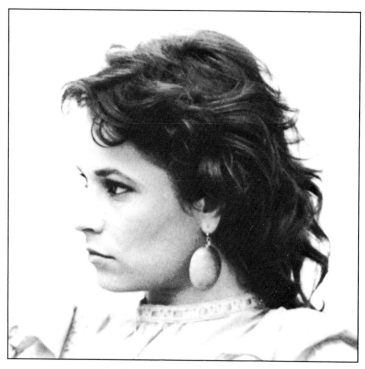

expense), is to make postcard-sized prints of one of your best shots, with your name, height, weight, and phone number printed at the bottom of the photo. This makes an impressive calling card, and many models leave these along with (or instead of) 8 x 10 prints since they believe it gives them an extra edge over the competition.

The kind of portfolio you should get is a plain black leather or vinyl zippered case. Portfolios that come with handles for carrying are the most practical for your needs. You can buy these in art supply stores and camera shops. Select a portfolio that is large enough to fit 8 x 10in (20 x 24cm) prints. It should also have clear plastic sleeves to protect the photos and hold them in place. Stick an adhesive label with your name, address and phone number on the inside flap of your book in case you should accidentally leave it somewhere. With your book in order, you will be ready to start scouting out employment opportunities, and visiting agencies.

## How to use your portfolio

You should aim for at least one professional working experience, such as a local fashion show, or newspaper fashion layout, before you start making the rounds of agencies. Remember that the more experience you can show the agencies, the more impressed they will be with your qualifications and natural enterprise.

If you are living in a small town, you should first contact charity organizations, to inquire about any fashion shows that they may sponsor in the near future. Also ring the fashion editor or women's page editor of the local newspaper and ask him or her about any shows given by department stores or boutiques that you may be able to model for. To be thorough, also contact the department stores and boutiques direct. Always remember to leave (or send) a photo of yourself with everyone you speak to — they may telephone you soon after with a job offer. When you get your first job, whether it is show modelling or informal, department store modelling, try to have someone there to shoot a roll of black and white pictures of you. Select the best one and put it in your book.

If you happen to live in a large city, there are a number of places you can contact and leave your photos. Start with newspapers, city-oriented weekly magazines; department stores, hair salons and boutiques. To prevent yourself from missing any business calls, you should consider buying a telephone-answering machine.

Another avenue you should explore is the young women's glossy magazine market. Send your photograph (and a stamped, self-addressed envelope) to the editorial department of these magazines. Include a brief covering letter informing them of your modelling experience, and current scholastic status — whether or not you are at school or college. Do not say, 'I have always wanted to be a model and that is why I am writing to you...' Be professional and state that you are committed to pursuing a career in modelling. The letter is just an informative courtesy; your picture will speak for itself.

Local beauty contests are also considered to be excellent opportunities for aspiring models, since they often promote their winners to national level. Needless to say, if you have won your local beauty contest, you will have achieved a certain celebrity status that you can probably cash in on. Use your imagination and create your own opportunities.

Finally, if you are in a big city, there is one more area to explore for possible modeling jobs: advertising agencies. Find out which ones do major print and/or television campaigns that require models. Because advertising photography often appears in several regional publications — and sometimes national ones — you should make the effort to get your photograph into the

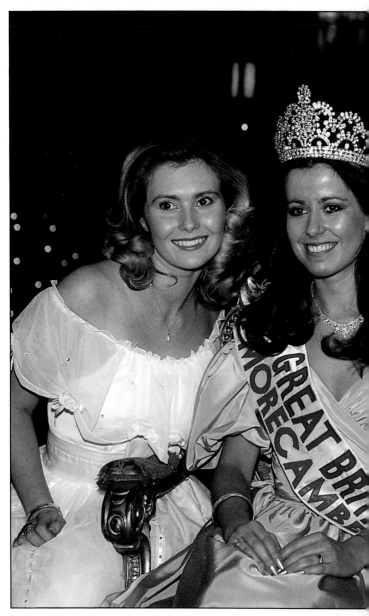

hands of an agency art director. Ask receptionists at the agencies for the correct spellings of the art directors' names. You should send them a personal business letter, rather than an off-putting form letter beginning with, 'Dear Sir/Madam...' Follow up your letters and photographs with a telephone call a week later. Ask the people who have received your material whether you could call in next week to show them your portfolio. If they tell you they are not interested, try to be as gracious as possible, and contact another agency. Once you have done a few freelance jobs, you will feel confident enough to approach a modeling agency. But first you should know what a modeling agency does, and what you should expect one to do for you.

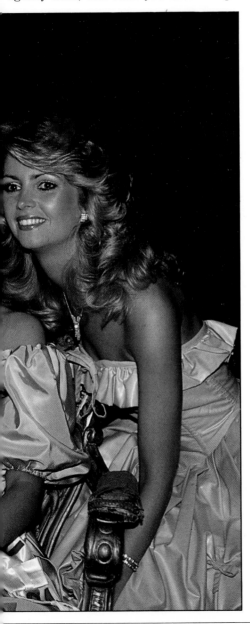

*Winning a local beauty contest is a good way to start a career in modeling. You may be promoted to national level, thus acquiring a certain celebrity status. Here the winner of the Miss Great Britain contest is pictured with the two runners-up.*

# PHOTO SESSIONS

The number of people working on a photo session — and the duration of the shoot — are determined by the type of job. Personnel for a magazine layout shoot at Francesco Scavullo's photo studios would include: models, a fashion editor and stylist, two studio assistants, a studio manager, as well as two freelance studio assistants. There would also be a hairstylist and makeup artist. Scavullo shoots as many as six to eight pages of fashion photographs a day, including magazine cover shots, and the studio's work day runs from about 9am to 6pm. Hair and makeup can sometimes take as long as 30 minutes for each set-up, so you should expect plenty of waiting in every shoot. Some models read; other pass the time in conversation with clients or colleagues.

A catalog shoot is often arranged on a strict timetable, as the art director plans specific situations with coordinated clothes to be photographed together. Most catalogs show models who are posed in rather standard formats, although this does not make catalog work any easier than other types of modeling. On the contrary, a day-long shoot for a department store's seasonal catalog can require the services of all of the people mentioned above, in addition to clothes ironers, set builders, film changers, one or more art directors, the department store's fashion coordinator, and makeup and hair assistants. On this kind of shoot, a model may be given up to 14 different outfits to wear, and will probably be asked to change her makeup and hair at least four times, for variety. A look into the contents of Lyne Pedola's catalog session work-bag will give you a good idea of the transformations that a professional model must be prepared for in the course of a catalog photo session:

- Several shades of panty hose, from sheer to black
- Nude, beige and white-colored half and full slips
- Nude and beige all-in-ones and bras
- Bust pads in three different sizes
- Foundations and face powders in shades ranging from translucent to beige
- A palette of lipstick shades
- A palette of eyeshadows
- Three different earth-toned nail polish colors eyeliners
- Powder puffs and sponges
- A lotion makeup remover
- Three different earth-toned nail polish colors
- Clear nail polish

*If shooting in far-flung locations, be sure to take basic essentials with you, such as your preferred brands of powder and eye makeup remover, as they may not be available locally.*

Remember that you won't always have to carry as many cosmetics around with you as Lyne did on this particular day. Most photographic studios and backstage areas of fashion shows stock cosmetics in the most commonly used color ranges, and, if a makeup artist is at your shoot or show, he or she will bring everything that is needed. Your booking agent will advise you about specific makeup or clothing requests before any shoot, anyway, so there should never be any doubts about what make-up you require. If you are going on location for a shoot, however, you should take everything that you may possibly need for the particular fashion you are modeling. You don't want to be stranded in the middle of a suburban golf course without a slip to wear under a clingy silk dress, for example. And if you are lucky enough to be shooting in far-flung locations, such as the French Virgin Islands or North Africa, you must be sure that you have got your preferred brands of powder and eye makeup remover because you may not be able to find them locally.

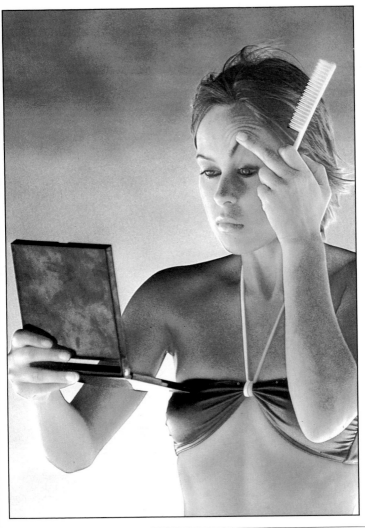

# LOCATION SHOOTING

Some models like to travel as much as possible and so make this preference known to their agencies. However, it is a lucky model who flies around the world for her bookings, and you should not expect to be considered for location assignments unless you have got some sound photo credits to your name, in national magazines, catalogues or advertising campaigns.

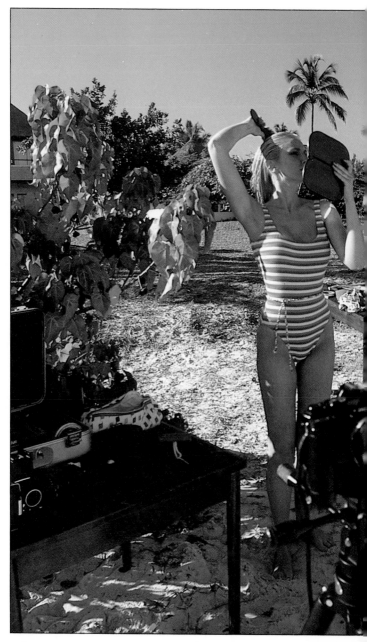

It is generally acknowledged in the industry that anything can go wrong on location, and often does. Such accidents as a model falling off a horse and ripping an expensive couture dress, or a sudden rainstorm drenching an entire crew and damaging the equipment, have been known to happen. More mundane problems include: waiting for cloudy skies to brighten; doing wardrobe changes out in the open; or malfunctioning bulbs and wiring. The most important thing to remember when anything goes wrong is that it's useful experience and a chance for you to show your professionalism.

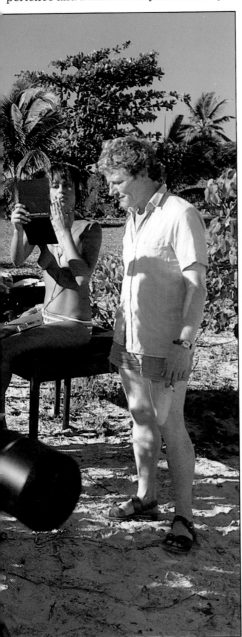

*Anything can go wrong on location — particularly with the weather or the equipment. But whatever happens, a model can prove her professionalism by showing she can cope in any situation.*

# MODELING AGENCIES

A modeling agency is in business to find work for its models by selling its services for fees that are determined by the nature of the job. Some agencies specialize in particular fields: television commercial modeling, photographic print modeling, or show modeling. An agency takes a percentage of the fees you earn in exchange for promoting you to their clients and sending you for interviews with potential employers. Once you are affiliated to an agency, all your business will be conducted by and through it.

When a client decides that he or she wants you for a job, the arrangements are handled by your booker. This person is responsible for negotiating your fees, billing the clients and collecting your fees. Usually, the first assignments a booker coordinates for a new model are test shoots with rising fashion photographers who have good relationships with the agencies. The reasons for doing this are quite practical: to get more good shots for the model's book, to get photographers' viewpoints about how the model works and what her strengths and weaknesses are, and to give the model more professional experience.

A good agency will devote time to personal consultation with their models, working with them on developing an improved self-awareness and attitude, as well as discussing the feedback they get from photographers and clients about the model's conduct during photo sessions or assignments. Nikki Gentile, of the Foster Fell Agency in New York, holds classes every Saturday for newly signed models. Formerly a print model with Wilhelmina Agency, one of New York's largest and most prestigious, Nikki explains, 'Unless you're a star model, you can't necessarily expect a lot of individual attention from a big agency. Their staff may handle close to two hundred models, and this is an important fact to be aware of when you're starting out and need guidance . . . A smaller agency can sometimes groom you and motivate you into becoming a much more experienced and professional model than a busy, top agency can. But all of this aside, I really believe that seventy-five per cent of your success ultimately has to do with your personality. You've got to be serious about your go-sees, you must always look and act like a professional, and you've got to be extremely committed. If I sign a model and groom her for six months and nothing's resulted from her test shoots or go-sees, then this is a pretty good indication that she's not going to work out in the long run. Six months is enough for both parties to see whether she's right for the business, and this is why I'm not particularly eager to sign models for long term contracts. Also, for certain types of models, like petites, it pays to be a freelancer, as there is not an overwhelming need for them in the market.'

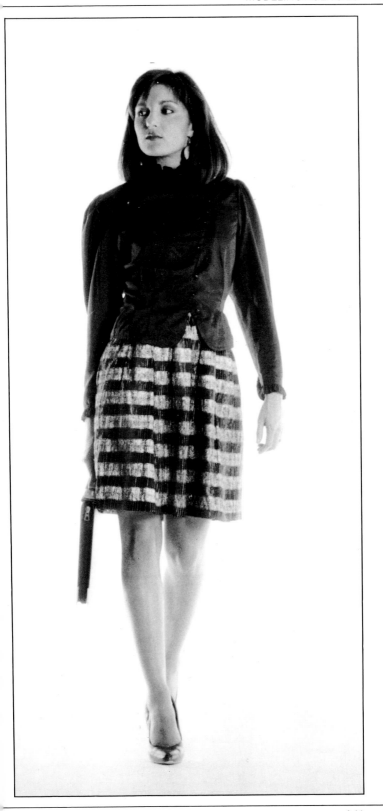

## How to get an interview with an agency

Most agencies hold interviews at certain times or on certain days of the week for would-be models. To make an appointment, ring them and explain that you are a new model. Tell them your height and your dress size, state your name clearly and ask for an appointment to show someone your book. If your body statistics are within the agency's preferred range, then you can expect to be given an appointment at once. For efficiency's sake, line up two appointments a day with the agencies in your town, and then prepare yourself thoroughly for inspection.

First decide what you are going to wear, and be sure that every article of clothing is in perfect condition. Never wear trousers to an interview, and save yourself the embarrassment of wearing over-dressy, formal clothes. You should select a simple dress, or a classically-styled blouse and skirt. Coordinate these with a plain-colored blazer or sweater. Wear medium-heeled shoes, or sandals if it is summer-time. Try to be as subtle with your make-up as possible. The people who screen models at agencies are experts at imagining how a face will look with dramatic colors and effects. Make it easy for them to see the natural beauty of your face, and save your new 'fire-engine' red lipstick for a more suitable occasion. Wear your hair styled simply and naturally; it should be clean and well-conditioned. Always be sure that your hands are in good condition if you have an important interview the following day. You may also want to consider having a facial.

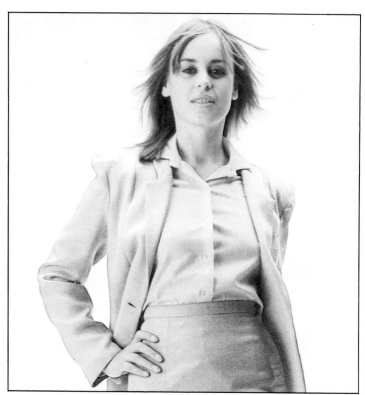

# How to handle agency interviews

Answer all questions with a calm, matter-of-fact attitude. Even if you have had no paid working experience, present yourself as seriously as you can. Agencies are constantly signing up models who have never worked professionally; they will not hold any lack of experience against you. Play it cool with your interviewer and let him or her study the contents of your book in silence. Do not be offended if the agency tells you to come back when you have lost some weight — they are only exercising professional judgement and obviously believe you have some potential. Take their advice and drop your weight by exercising more and eating less. When you return, they will be impressed by your persistence, and may decide to take you on.

If you are rejected outright, do not allow yourself to take it personally. Rejection is a commonplace ingredient in a model's life. It could be that the agency approves of your brown-haired, green-eyed looks, but if they are already managing 20 girls of the same type, they will not be particularly anxious to give you a contract. If you really think that you have a chance, then do not give up easily. A rejection is not necessarily a final decision. Times change, and certain types of looks move in and out of fashion. Your particular looks may swing into vogue *after* you have been around to several agencies. This is why it is a good idea to try making new appointments six months to a year after your initial interview. Show them some new and improved test shots and hope for the best.

When concluding your meetings, always leave your photograph with the person who interviewed you. It is possible that the agency will decide they want you after all, or perhaps a particular assignment will arise that calls for a model with precisely your looks. If you should be turned down by every agency you visit, then perhaps you should re-evaluate your qualifications and reasons for wanting to be a model. If you are still convinced that you have the requisite looks and talent, then you must test with as many photographers as possible until you produce some slides and prints that give your beliefs some substance. Try talking to photographers and agency personnel about where you are going wrong, listen carefully to what they have to say, and then reassess the situation.

*To create a good impression at an interview wear a simple, smart outfit, a small amount of make-up and your hair in a natural style.*

## Questions to ask an agency

If an agency decides to take you on, get definite answers to the following questions before signing a contract with them:

- Will I get paid on a monthly or weekly basis, or only when the clients pay up?
- What is your procedure for negotiating, billing and collecting my fees from clients? How much do you take from my fee as your commission?
- Will I be able to borrow money from you if and when business is slow?
- How much do you charge clients if they cancel one of my bookings? Will I get paid my regularly hourly rate if a client cancels?
- What sort of model will you promote me as? Catalogue, high fashion, advertising? Can you promote me for various fields at once?
- When can I expect my first booking from you?
- Will you be able to advance the cost of prints, slides and composites if I am short on funds?

If you are satisfied with the answers to these questions, your booker will then tell you how often to report in over the phone, what your starting rates will be, and other essential information. Your agency will incorporate your photo on their 'headsheet', a brochure with photos of every model currently represented by them, with the models' vital information listed underneath. As well as scheduling test shoots for you, after you have done some photographic work, your agency will start assembling your 'composite', which is a card, or brochure, of several of your best shots, as well as your measurements; eye and hair color, and special attributes, such as 'excellent hands and legs'. Agencies usually expect you to pay for the cost of printing your composite, but, as this can be quite expensive, they often advance the money to a promising new model.

If your booker is arranging a steady stream of jobs for you in catalog and other types of photographic modeling, but your professional goal is to model in high fashion shows, do not complain about the nature of your work. You are gaining invaluable experience. After six months of these jobs, you have a better chance of getting show modeling work than you did before. Now is the time to discuss your ambitions with your agent, because you have both professional skills and some authentic bargaining power. Always assume responsibility for your career making the most of every opportunity. Success in one field of the business will be a passport to another.

## How to find an agency

The final section of this book contains a comprehensive list of modeling schools and agencies in America and England. Although every attempt has been made to include only the best agencies in the country, do research *any* agency before you consider signing with them. Check with your local Consumer's Union, speak with models under contract to the agency, and keep looking until you find one that seems right for you.

# Keeping track of expenses

Ford model Lyne Pedola says that she saves and files all her professional receipts, such as bills from her beautician and hairdresser, because she can deduct part of her financial outgoings from her taxes. Other models' deductibles include: taxi receipts, phone calls made in relation to work, and part of the cost of an answering machine or answering service. Be sure to keep track of all of the above, as it will save you money in the long run. Your agency will probably be able to recommend a reliable accountant who is experienced in handling models' taxes and expenses.

**Model release form** *It is important to establish a clear arrangement with photographers and agencies. Many agencies do not have contracts, but the model release form (above) should be explained to a model before a session. Once she has signed the form she has given the photographer permission to use the pictures.*

| AD. AGENCY/PHOTOG. | 1 |
| MODEL AGENT | 2 |
| MODEL | 3 |

**This is a generic model release form. Although formats vary, the information contained is always the same as below.**

NAME OF PHOTOGRAPHER

NAME OF *ADVERTISING AGENCY/CLIENT

PRODUCT, SERVICE OR PURPOSE

NEGATIVE SERIES NO.          ORDER NO.          DATE

In consideration of the sum of          and any other sums which may become due to me under the above Associations' current "Terms, conditions and standards for the engagement of professional models in still photography", and conditionally upon due payment of the aforesaid sums and the undertaking of the *Advertising Agency/Client/Photographer given below, I permit the *Advertising Agency/Client/Photographer and its licensees or assignees to use the photograph(s) referred to above and/or drawings therefrom and any other reproductions or adaptations thereof either complete or in part, alone or in conjunction with any wording and/or drawings solely and exclusively for:

- ★ **EDITORIAL**
- ★ **EXPERIMENTAL**
- ★ **PR**
- ★ **PRESS ADVERTISING**
- ★ **POSTER ADVERTISING** (4 sheet upwards)
- ★ **DISPLAY MATERIAL AND POSTERS** (under 4 sheet)
- ★ **PACKAGING**

in relation to the above product, service, or purpose

- ★ **IN THE UNITED KINGDOM**
- ★ **IN EUROPE**
- ★ **WORLDWIDE**

*MODELS MUST DELETE IF NOT APPLICABLE

I understand that such copyright material shall be deemed to represent an imaginary person unless agreed, in writing, by my agent or myself.
I understand that I do not own the copyright of the photograph(s).

* I am over 18 years of age.

NAME (in capitals)

SIGNATURE OF MODEL

ADDRESS/AGENT

DATE          WITNESS

*Models who are under 18 years of age must produce evidence of consent by their parent or guardian.*

In accepting the above release the *Advertising Agency/Client/Photographer undertakes that

the copyright material shall only be used in accordance with the terms of the release.

*MODELS MUST DELETE IF NOT APPLICABLE          PRINTED IN 1984

# 5
# TRAVELING IN STYLE

## THE TRAVEL BAG

## ARRIVING REFRESHED

## EXERCISE

## EATING OUT

## HEALTH CARE

## JETLAG

*E*veryone who travels faces the
same problems: what to pack,
how to occupy the time in transit, how to arrive
refreshed, how to stick to a reasonable
diet, and follow beauty care and exercise routines
in unfamiliar environments. Some people
never master this delicate balancing act
and invariably return from business trips or
vacations looking out of shape
and feeling mentally and physically tired. With a
little planning, you can organize your
health and beauty regime to fit in with your
traveling. There's no reason why
you cannot feel your best while you are away, and
the following chapter provides some
key answers to how you can maintain optimum
health and wellbeing wherever you are
and whatever you are doing.

# THE TRAVEL BAG

Regardless of the contents of your travel wardrobe — casual and business clothes, sporty vacation wear or evening gowns — you should be sure to pack practical items such as a portable steam iron for smoothing out wrinkled garments, a pocket-sized sewing kit for quick repairing of hems or buttons and, if you are wearing dark clothes, an adhesive roller brush that picks up lint and stray hairs. If you are taking any shoes or boots that need regular applications of oil or polish, then you should pack some of these too.

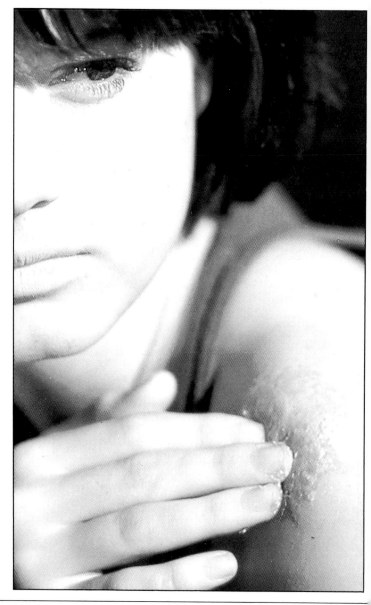

Apart from the cosmetics that you use every day, you should also consider including a few items that will be particularly useful in the climate that you're visiting. Products such as rich moisturizers, mineral water spray and medicated lip balm are useful for protecting your face and body in cold, damp or hot climates. If you are heading south, or taking a beach vacation, you will definitely want to assemble some or all of the following: a toner, astringent, or clarifying lotion, mineral water spray, lip balm that contains a sun protection factor, tanning lotion that is strong enough to keep you from burning; an overall moisturizer for applying when you come out of the sun, a pair of dark sunglasses to protect your eyes, and hair clips, headbands or scarves to keep your hair off your face.

---

### THE PORTABLE BEAUTY KIT

Here is a suggested shortlist for your traveling beauty kit:
- Daily makeup products, such as foundation, powder, blusher, mascara, eyeshadows.
- A cleansing soap or cream; eye makeup remover pads or lotion.
- An astringent or alcohol-free toner; cotton cosmetic pads and cotton swabs for makeup and eye makeup removal.
- Your moisturizer, hand cream, foot cream or night cream.
- Emery boards, nail clippers, hairstyling brush and any other utensils, such as tweezers or eyelash curlers, that you regularly use.
- Hairpins, ties, headbands.
- An effective indigestion remedy that will settle an upset stomach, relieve heartburn and other common digestive ailments. Tablets are perfect for travelers, as they take up little space in a suitcase or handbag.
- A small mineral water spray for freshening your face in the morning, setting your makeup and hairstyle, and for misting your face after moisturizing at night.
- Sachets of shampoo and conditioner; hairspray and styling gel if you use them.
- Shaving cream and a razor.
- Toothpaste, toothbrush, dental floss.
- Nail polish and acetone-free nail polish remover, if you use them.
- Perfume, cologne or eau de toilette — whichever one suits the circumstances.
- Any medication you regularly take or think you may need, such as motion sickness pills.
- If you take vitamins daily, put some in a small pillbox.

---

*When you are traveling remember to pack creams for applying before and after sunbathing and any medication you need.*

## Arriving refreshed

When traveling by plane, there are a few important steps you can take to protect your skin and general health during the flight. Although plane travel can be relatively comfortable, the pressurized cabins, stale air and lack of humidity in the plane can trigger such reactions as dry and itchy skin, extreme thirst, constipation, puffy bloodshot eyes and earaches. To minimize any discomfort you may experience during travelling, New York make-up artist Patrick Denis offers the following advice:

● Pack some chewing gum in your purse and chew during take-off to relieve your ears of sudden changes in pressure that can lead to earaches.

● Wear very little makeup on the plane (if you must, wear mascara and eyeliner only). Wear plenty of moisturizer on your face and reapply it every few hours. Also rub moisturizer into hands and elbows if they have a tendency to become dry.

● Do not eat the meals served on planes. Besides being low in nutritional value, they are invariably processed foods, laden with salt and preservatives, guaranteed to cause water retention and slow digestion. Bring your own food, like carrot sticks, nuts, cheese, raisins or a sandwich. Also bring a bottle of sodium-free soda water or flat mineral water, as many planes do not serve these. Drinking a glass of water or fruit juice every hour will replenish the fluids that your body loses as a result of the plane's dry environment.

● Do not drink too much alcohol during the flight. This will make you very dehydrated, and can often result in splitting headaches, if you are on a long flight and have more than a couple of drinks. Also remember that the high altitudes and pressure inside the plane make you more susceptible to the effects of alcohol.

● Pack a bottle of saline solution eyedrops for bloodshot, tired or itchy eyes.

● If your face and eyes are puffy after the flight, make a compress of a face cloth and cool water. Lay it across your face for twenty minutes. Alternatively, take teabags that have been briefly dipped in lukewarm water and place one on each eye. Lie down and leave them on for 15 minutes. This will reduce puffiness and dark circles effectively.

*To combat the dehydrating effects of plane journeys, avoid alcohol and pre-packaged meals, and wear very little (if any) makeup.*

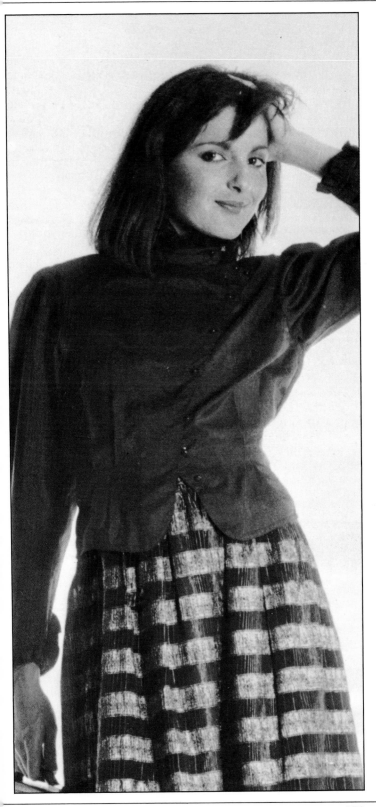

# EXERCISE

Long, confined plane, train or car trips can be physically tiring. Bad circulation, stiffness in joints and muscles and overall tension are just some of the familar signs of traveling, whether for business or pleasure. Beginning with exercises you can do while seated in a plane, train or car seat, there are several beneficial workout routines that can be readily integrated into your traveling schedules.

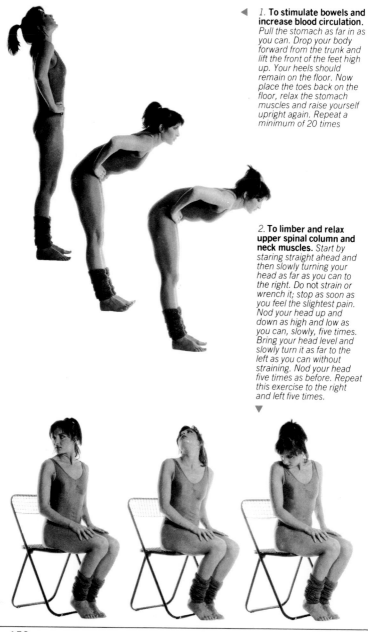

◄ *1.* **To stimulate bowels and increase blood circulation.** *Pull the stomach as far in as you can. Drop your body forward from the trunk and lift the front of the feet high up. Your heels should remain on the floor. Now place the toes back on the floor, relax the stomach muscles and raise yourself upright again. Repeat a minimum of 20 times*

*2.* **To limber and relax upper spinal column and neck muscles.** *Start by staring straight ahead and then slowly turning your head as far as you can to the right. Do not strain or wrench it; stop as soon as you feel the slightest pain. Nod your head up and down as high and low as you can, slowly, five times. Bring your head level and slowly turn it as far to the left as you can without straining. Nod your head five times as before. Repeat this exercise to the right and left five times.*

▼

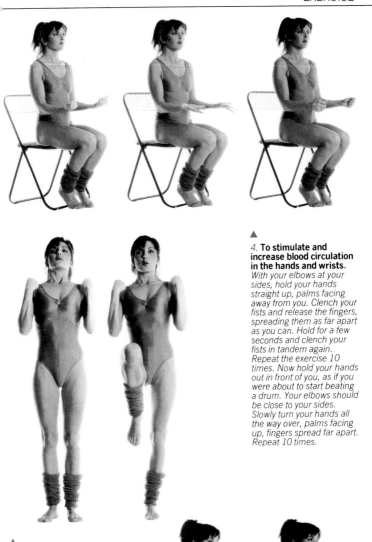

**4. To stimulate and increase blood circulation in the hands and wrists.** *With your elbows at your sides, hold your hands straight up, palms facing away from you. Clench your fists and release the fingers, spreading them as far apart as you can. Hold for a few seconds and clench your fists in tandem again. Repeat the exercise 10 times. Now hold your hands out in front of you, as if you were about to start beating a drum. Your elbows should be close to your sides. Slowly turn your hands all the way over, palms facing up, fingers spread far apart. Repeat 10 times.*

**3. To increase blood circulation.** *Hold arms up to your front so that the inside of your fists are level with and facing your shoulders. Your elbows should be at your sides. Now lift the left and right knees alternately up to touch the opposite elbow. Do this 10 times in each direction.*

**5. To relieve tension and swelling in ankles and increase blood flow to the feet.** *Pick up one foot and roll your ankle in a circular movement. Your calf and thigh should remain perfectly motionless — only your foot and ankle should move. Repeat 15 times in each direction and repeat the exercise with the other foot.*

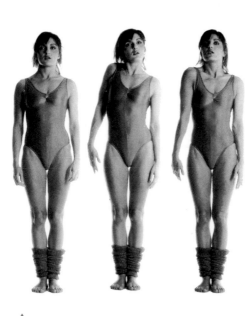

1. *Lean back on your elbows and alternately bring one knee to the chest while the other leg is held straight out, toes flexed upwards. Your leg and stomach muscles will benefit from this movement; so will your circulation. Repeat at least 10 times.*
2. *Leaning back on your elbows, alternately flex and point your feet, extending each leg as far as it can go. Repeat at least 10 times with each leg.*
3. *Sitting upright in the tub, alternately lift your legs 3in (7.5cm) and hold this position for three seconds. Repeat at least 10 times with each leg.*

6. **To relax neck, shoulder and back muscles.** *Staring straight ahead, rotate your shoulders forward in slow, rhythmic circles. Repeat 10 times and then roll shoulders backward 10 times. Roll your right shoulder in both directions 10 times and repeat the process with the left shoulder.*

7. **To relax feet and increase blood flow in feet and ankles.** *Remove your shoes and alternately flex and relax your toes 15 times. Do this with both feet.*

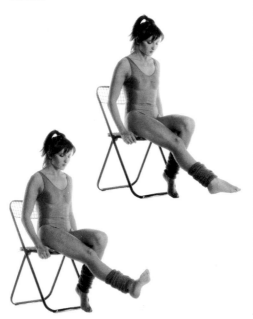

# BATHTUB EXERCISES

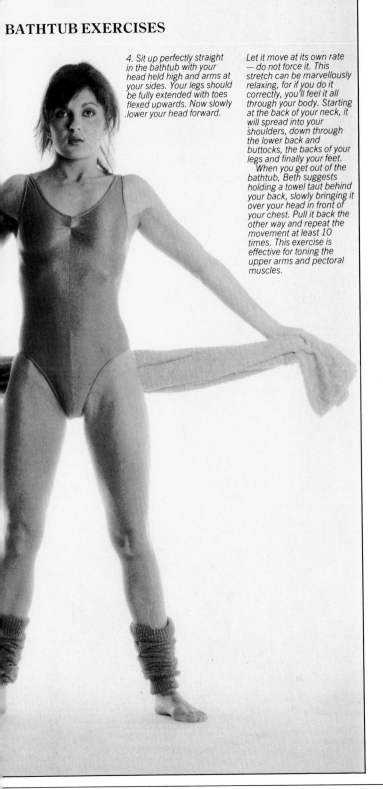

4. Sit up perfectly straight in the bathtub with your head held high and arms at your sides. Your legs should be fully extended with toes flexed upwards. Now slowly lower your head forward.

Let it move at its own rate — do not force it. This stretch can be marvellously relaxing, for if you do it correctly, you'll feel it all through your body. Starting at the back of your neck, it will spread into your shoulders, down through the lower back and buttocks, the backs of your legs and finally your feet.

When you get out of the bathtub, Beth suggests holding a towel taut behind your back, slowly bringing it over your head in front of your chest. Pull it back the other way and repeat the movement at least 10 times. This exercise is effective for toning the upper arms and pectoral muscles.

## Hotel Workouts

There are several hotelroom workouts and exercise options
that you can follow to maintain your level of fitness while you
are away from home. For instance, if your room has a television,
you can work out with an early morning exercise program on
one of the local or national television stations. Almost every city
broadcasts one between the hours of six and nine in the morning. Pack some comfortable exercise clothes and sneakers and
you will be ready to start the day with a half hour of serious exercise. You might also want to consider traveling with an exercise
cassette. Aerobic dance, yoga, isometric exercises — these are
all available in stores around the country. If you buy several different ones, it is possible to have a very diverse workout
schedule, and you'll suffer none of the boredom of repetitious
exercise routines. Cassette players are now being manufac-
tured in highly compact sizes (some are as small as a bar of
soap), so they won't take up much room in your luggage.

If your regular fitness routine involves lifting weights or using exercise machines, print and television model Beth Rubino
offers the following suggestions for keeping fit in your hotelroom:

● Pack a retractable chinning bar for exercising your upper
body. These bars fit into most standard suitcases and the rubber
suction pads at either end of the bar fix them to a door frame for
exercising.

● To exercise the rest of your body, you can perform the exercises on the following pages. These are chosen because they
work the muscle areas that are quick to lose firmness, such as
the upper arm (triceps), the buttocks, the abdominals, and the
lower abdominals.

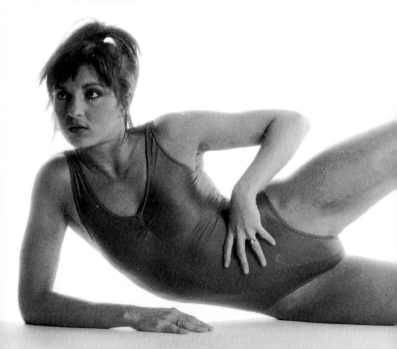

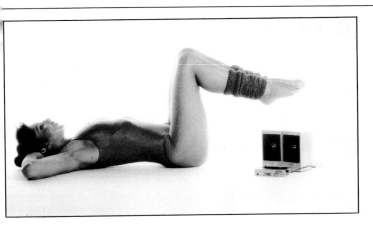

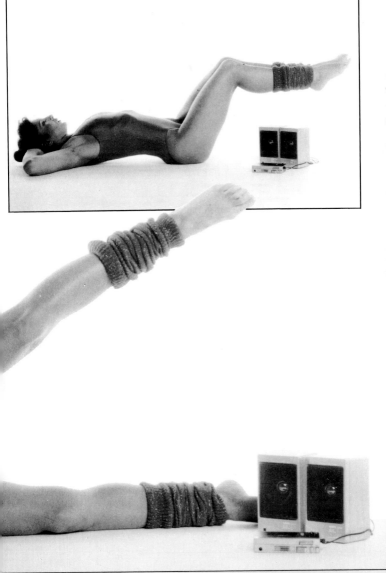

*1.* **For the upper arm and back.** *This is an invigorating pushup.* First, place two chairs, approximately the same height, about a body length apart. You may have to adjust this, as you will see. The chair seats should be facing each other. With your hands clasping the edges of one chair seat behind you, extend your arms to support your upper body. Now adjust the other chair so that your heels are resting on it. Your seat and legs should be an L-shape, with your legs extended straight out in front of you, your heels firmly planted on the other chair. Now you are ready to push up. You should do this exercise slowly and smoothly. Do not let yourself drop down quickly — lower and raise yourself steadily as you perform the pushup part of the exercise. A pushup always demands a proper breathing technique, so do remember to inhale as your body is going down and exhale as it rises up. Repeat a minimum of 10 times.

*2.* **For buttocks.** *Stand with your feet shoulder-width apart in front of a dresser or table, or any piece of furniture that you can hold onto with your hands at waist to chest height. Place a chair behind you. Grasp the dresser at the sides and hold your back straight. Lower your seat to the chair without sitting, and stand back up without leaning,*

letting the muscles of your thighs and buttocks lift you. Repeat a minimum of 15 times.

*3.* **Lower abdominal toning.** *Lie on your back with your hands under your buttocks. Lift both legs 6in (15cm) from the floor. Tuck your knees in towards your chest, then stretch your legs straight out again. Your feet and legs should never touch the floor as you repeat this for a minimum of 15 times.*

*4.* **Toning the back and waist.** *You need a sturdy door for this. Open it halfway, placing your feet firmly on either side of it at the bottom, heels together. Grasp the door knobs on either side and lean back, bending at the waist. Now, without moving your legs, pull yourself straight up and touch the door with your chest. Your bowed waist and chest stay on the same plane as you approach and touch the door. Then lean back slowly again, letting your arms extend fully. The purpose of this exercise is to make your back do all the work. If the muscles in your arms are straining, you are not doing it right. Keep trying until you feel your back pulling your body in and out. Repeat 10 times.*

*5.* **Toning abdominal muscles.** *Find a solid piece of furniture — a desk, table, dresser or bed frame will do. Sit on the floor with your legs bent and your feet underneath a desk*

drawer, for example. Place your hands on the small of your back, fingers interlocked at the level of your waistline. Your palms should face out. Lower yourself backward until your palms touch the floor and raise yourself up again. Repeat a minimum of 10 times. This exercise is also good for easing tension in the lower back.

*6.* **Limbering and toning shoulders.** *Stand in a doorway with feet shoulder width apart. Make fists and press the backs of your hands against either side of the doorway. Push outward and upward, holding for four seconds at peak height and tension. Relax and repeat a minimum of 10 times.*

If Beth's exercises don't appeal to you, you should check on what kind of fitness facilities are available to you before you go. Your hotel or vacation spot may have a swimming pool and running track or these facilities may exist nearby. If this is the case you will want to take your swimsuit or running gear with you. Another excellent exercise alternative is a skipping rope. You can have a brisk aerobic workout in your room in the morning and/or at night while you watch television or listen to music.

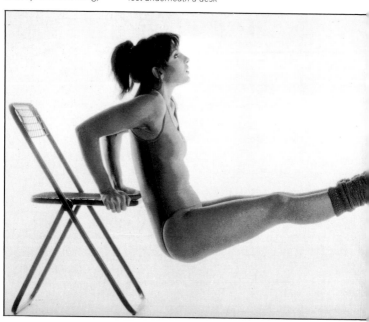

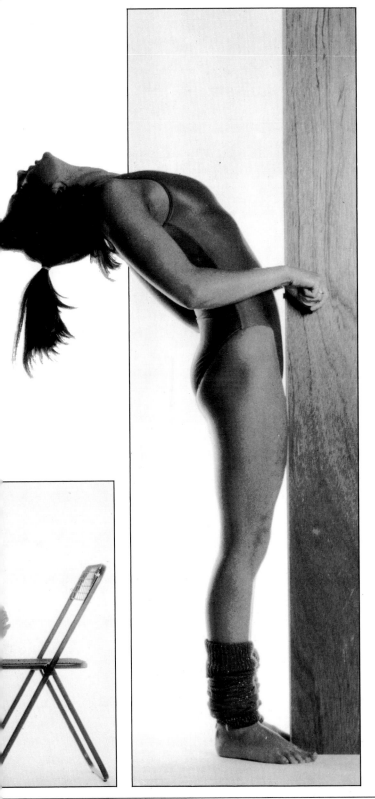

# EATING OUT

It has gradually dawned on hotel and restaurant owners around the world that a great many of us see the vital connections between diet and health. More and more of us are no longer interested in rich, high-calorie foods because of the various health complications that they can trigger — being overweight the most obvious. Just because you are on vacation, or going out for 'working' dinners, there is no reason why you cannot eat sensible, high energy, low calorie meals. Even the Queen Elizabeth II, the grande dame of luxury ocean liners, offers nutritious, 'dieter's' menus in all of its dining rooms. Healthy diet trends aside, what can you do to keep your eating habits on an even keel during your trip?

Anne Soorikian, a New York beauty editor and veteran of countless business luncheons and food-filled vacations, believes self-control is all-important. 'You should know what you can eat and what will make you gain weight. You've got to realize that what you eat may change your shape for the better — or worse. If you go ahead and eat a heavy meal plus dessert without first admitting to yourself that it will cost you 3lb (1.3kg), then you're never going to maintain your ideal weight. Other self-control measures that are also important are eliminating nervous snacking. If you must eat something, eat half a cup of strawberries, or a salad with no dressing. Sometimes when we're out of our customary surroundings we're tempted to eat more, but this is no excuse. You've just got to tell yourself that you can get through the day without relying on food. Another pitfall that many people are prone to is overeating because someone is treating them to a delicious dinner. The occasion could be business or pleasure, but if this type of eating pattern continues over a period of time, you could gain a noticeable amount of weight. The only way to avoid losing your shape is by exercising your self-control at every meal, and between them, too.'

But what can you do if you are seated in a restaurant whose menu boasts one rich, taboo entree after another and all you really want is a low fat, low calorie dish like grilled sole with lemon? The answer is simple. Order it. Never hesitate to ask for something made to order. This includes vegetable dishes, as well. Ask your waiter or waitress if the vegetables are prepared with butter or oil. If it is possible to have them steamed or broiled along with your main dish, then this is a good solution for someone who is watching their weight. If all the desserts on the menu are in the forbidden, high-calorie zone, simply order coffee or tea or some fresh fruit.

If you don't want to eat as carefully as this all the time you are away, you can afford to break your diet every now and then without putting on too much weight. Beth Rubino's dieting discipline will work in these circumstances: watch what you eat for the first three days of the week and stick to your usual restrictions. On the fourth day, eat one meal, preferably lunch, that is a treat — a deviation from your normal intake. For the next two days, eat very carefully again, remaining diet-conscious and, on the seventh day, have a fiesta — eat anything and everything you've craved all week. 'This system allows you to go crazy with food, only within reason', Beth explains. 'You don't feel bad about eating a lot at the end of the week and, as a result, it's easy to be disciplined for the rest of the time. You also get to exercise self-control in a very controlled situation. You know what the rules are and you also know that you can maintain your weight and still have all the food you want for one day of the week.' Other models interviewed for this book offered similar strategies for keeping their figures. They are proof that it is possible to enjoy your food and still stay slim.

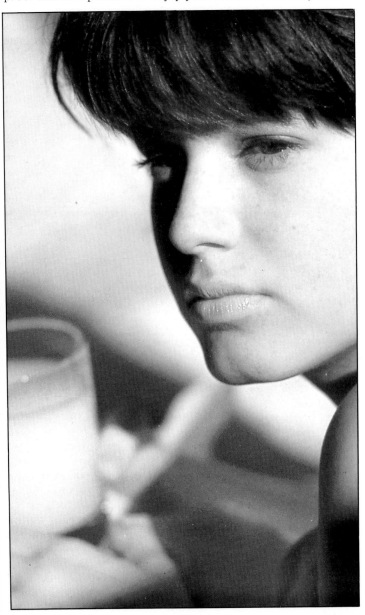

# HEALTH CARE

No chapter on caring for your health and beauty while traveling would be complete without advice on how to cope with the food and water in a foreign land. Very often the water supply will contain minerals and bacteria that are more highly concentrated than those found in your normal drinking water. Be warned

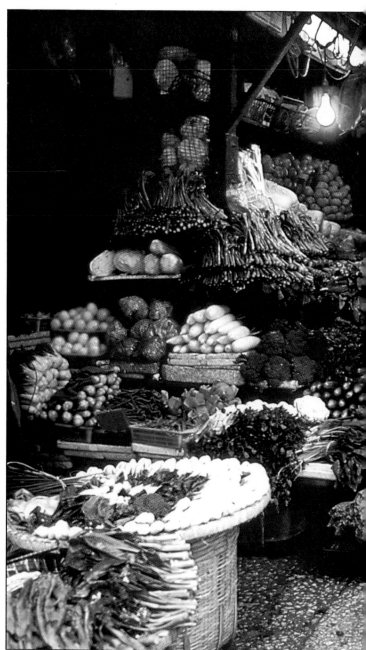

that, especially in the tropics, the incidence of food and water contamination is very high. If traveling to the tropics or a developing country, it is wise to get a gamma-globulin innoculation a week before you depart to prevent hepatitis. The stress of a long trip, combined with a new diet, and a change in your normal schedule can often trigger various digestive ailments. Traveler's diarrhoea (turista), abdominal cramps, constipation and vomiting are known to strike those vacationing in four star European hotels as well as visitors to India.

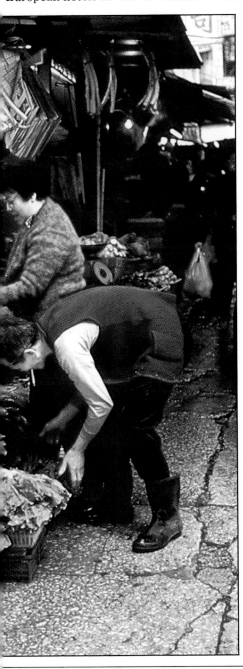

When working in faraway places, avoid fresh vegetables, locally produced dairy products and rare or raw meat and fish as these all carry a high risk of contamination. Do not eat any fruits except those with thick skins such as bananas, citrus fruits and melons.

# GOING ABROAD

| Disease | Risk Areas | Vaccination |
|---|---|---|
| **Yellow fever** | Africa, Central and South America | 1 injection at least 10 days before going abroad. Must be 2-week gap between this and polio. |
| **Cholera** | Africa, Asia, Middle East | 2 injections, 1 to 4 weeks apart |
| **Polio** | Everywhere, except Australia, New Zealand, Northern Europe, North America | Oral drops 3 doses, 4-8 weeks apart |
| **Typhoid** | 2 injections, 4-6 weeks apart | After 2nd injection, for 3 years |
| **Tetanus** | Everywhere | Course of 3 injections initially, then booster injection if at risk |
| **Infectious hepatitis** | Places where sanitation is primitive | No specific vaccine. 1 injection of immuno-globulin if in high risk area |

A good way of avoiding these illnesses is not to drink the tap water. This also applies to ice cubes, as they are frozen tap water. Stick to bottled mineral water or carbonated water, and use either of these for brushing your teeth, as a mouthful of water — unswallowed or swallowed — is enough to upset your whole system. Bottled sodas and beer are alright to drink, as are hot drinks made with boiled water.

Avoiding certain foods will also help ensure that you maintain your equilibrium when traveling. Foods that have a higher risk of contamination are fresh vegetables, locally produced dairy products, rare or raw meat, and fish. Do not sample food from street vendors — you don't know what sanitary measures were involved or how long the food has been sitting. Do not eat any fruits except those with thick skins, such as bananas, citrus fruit and melons. Restrict your diet to cooked fruits and vegetables, thoroughly cooked meats and dairy products from industrialized, commercial processors. Remember to follow these rules even if you are eating in someone's home, as your body is not as immune to the bacterial strains in local food. Gracefully decline when they offer cheese, fruit or salad, or any other dish that may upset your stomach.

All of these precautions aside, what should you do if you are stricken with any one of the illnesses previously mentioned?

| Period of cover | Reactions/notes |
| --- | --- |
| From 10 days after injection, for 10 years | Caution if allergic to eggs. Not given to children under 1 year old, or to pregnant women. Certificate needed. |
| 6 days after injection for 6 months | Certificate needed. NB Take care over hygiene as additional precaution. |
| Immediately after 3rd injection, for 3 years | |
| | |
| Immediately, for 5 years | |
| Immediately, for 4-6 months | Take care over hygiene as additional precaution. |

*Before you travel to far-away places, especially tropical or sub-tropical regions, check with your doctor whether you'll need immunization against diseases such as yellow fever, cholera, polio, typhoid, tetanus, malaria and smallpox. Once there, watch out for rabid animals; if you get bitten or scratched, seek medical help imme-diately. Be scrupulous about hygiene. Always wash your hands before eating, check that the water is safe to drink and avoid eating raw vegetables, unpeeled fruit, ice-cream, ice cubes, raw shellfish, underdone meat and fish and reheated food.*

Prepare for the possibility of sickness by packing some pre-scription remedies that treat diarrhoea, vomiting and stomach pains. If you visit your doctor before you leave, explaining what region you are travelling to, you will be prescribed some appro-priate medicine. If your illness does not subside in a day or two, or your symptoms become more severe, this could mean that water- or food-borne parasites are present in your body. Visit a doctor immediately and have your condition diagnosed and treated appropriately. Ask your doctor to give you a check-up when you return, just to make sure that the illness has com-pletely cleared up.

## Flying with a head cold

If you are suffering from a head cold, earache, or cold-related congestion, do not get on the plane. Most doctors strongly recommend that you postpone your flight until your health has cleared up. This is because people with colds and congestion have been known to suffer ear damage, extreme discomfort and sinus infection after a flight. If you have a mild cold with little congestion, you will be alright on the plane, but you should use a decongestant nasal spray before the plane takes off and lands. Chewing gum during the flight will keep your ears unplugged and make you feel more comfortable.

# JETLAG

For years, medical researchers have worked on a remedy for the tiring side-effects of jet plane travel. There is no miracle solution, but if you feel like experimenting with a new and popular diet that many doctors and travelers support, you may find that it lessens the physical toll of flights of three hours or more. The 'Anti-Jet Lag Diet' should be started three days before you leave on your trip as its purpose is to re-programme your system to a new environment and time zone.

*Day One*
Eat a high-protein breakfast of steak, eggs or liver. Tofu and scrambled eggs are also a good choice. Lunch should also be high in protein; have a meat or fish dish with lima beans, green beans or chick peas. Dinner shoud be high-carbohydrate, with bread, potatoes or pasta, starchy vegetables and a sweet dessert. Drink caffeine beverages *only* between the hours of 3pm and 5pm.

*Day Two*
Eat light meals: dry toast, clear soup, fruit, salads and fruit juice. Again, take no coffee or tea, except between 3pm and 5pm.

*Day Three*
Follow the menu plan for Day One.

*Day Four*
Follow the menu plan for Day Two. If you are travelling westwards only drink caffeine beverages in the morning, or between 6pm and 11pm if you are travelling eastwards. Once on board the plane, set your watch to the time it should be when you reach your destination. If the flight is a long one, sleep until breakfast time. While the other passengers doze on, eat a high protein breakfast for extra energy. Stay awake and walk up and down the aisles a few times; your body needs to be active. When you arrive, stay active and eat a high-protein lunch and high-carbohydrate dinner. You should awake refreshed and energetic the next morning, feeling none of the sluggishness that usually follows a long trip.

*On long-haul journeys, make sure you arrive refreshed by following the Anti Jet-Lag Diet outlined above. To get the right amount of sleep, drink coffee or tea in the morning when traveling west and between 6 and 11 p.m. when traveling east. Sleep until breakfast, eat a high-protein meal, then keep active by walking up and down the aisles a few times.*

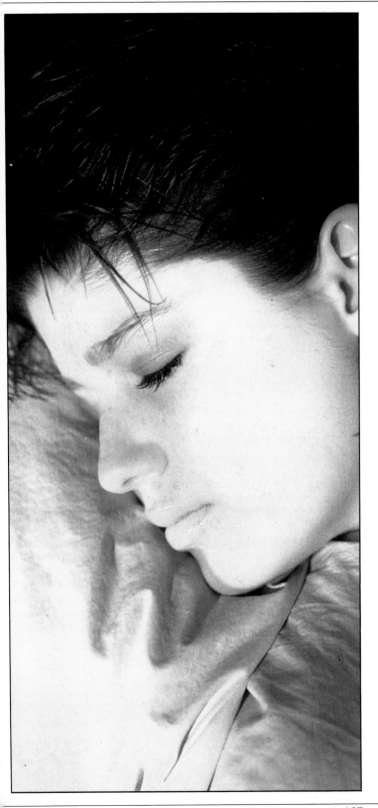

# BEAUTY TIPS

1.  Always wait for at least three hours before exercising if you have eaten a heavy meal or taken a hot bath. Wait half an hour after waking up from a night's sleep or a nap before exercising.

2.  The following low-calorie drinks are beneficial:
    *   Bottled mineral water with a citrus twist (page 26)
    *   Tomato juice
    *   Grapefruit juice
    *   Tea with lemon, no sugar

3.  Avocados are rich in oil and nutrients and help to keep your hair shiny and strong.

4.  Vitamin E oil (from a bottle or capsule) is an excellent skin conditioner. It clears up dry patches within hours and is especially gentle on sensitive areas.

5.  To reduce swelling of bruised areas: Finely grate a *yellow* apple (other kinds will not work). Make a compress by laying the grated apple between two squares of clean soft cotton or gauze. Hold this against the bruise for half an hour. The swelling should go down considerably after this application.

6.  To relieve sunburn: Place bags of camomile tea (lukewarm) on the affected area to act as a compress.

7.  To preserve a suntan: Facial scrubs or loofahs will brighten your tan by removing any dead skin that is dulling the glow. Don't worry about scrubbing off your tan — the only way it will fade is if you stay out of the sun.

8.  To relieve insect bites and stings: Wrap some crushed ice in clean gauze or cloth and hold this compress firmly against the affected area. Do not apply ice directly to the skin.

9.  The best way to clean your ears: Because wax lubricates and protects the delicate parts of the ear, specialists advise against the use of cotton swabs as they can pack the wax deeper and cause discomfort. Instead shampoo your hair often and the wax will dissolve. Alternatively wash your ears with a cotton washcloth. Use cotton swabs for drying the outer ear only.

10. The best way to shave legs and underarms: Choose a manual razor with a single-edged blade to reduce the number of nicks and cuts. Use non-medicated, non-aerosol and non-scented shaving cream. Shaving in the shower or tub is advisable as it softens the hair and skin first. Before applying shaving cream, work up a good lather with a rich moisturizing soap bar. Rinse and apply a generous amount of shaving cream. Never apply deodorant after shaving underarms as this can cause irritation.

11. To soothe red or itchy eyes: Try to avoid chemical eye drop solutions — they tend to provide temporary relief only and in some cases they dry out the eyes. A saline solution is best or simply splash cool water in and around the eyes.

12. To remove a particle from your eye: Do not rub the eye. The safest way to deal with this is by dousing your eye with cool water — tap water is fine. Saline solution sold for contact lenses is the best treatment for this problem as it squirts a stream of

fluid directly into the eye. If you have followed this treatment and your eye continues to feel irritated, then you should see a doctor as soon as possible.

13.  To make eyelashes look longer: Lightly powder your eyelashes with baby powder or translucent face powder. Stroke on a coat of mascara. Powder again and stroke on another coat.

14.  To make eyeshadow last longer: Eyeshadow cream 'fixers' which are applied before shadow, help your makeup to go on smoothly and blend in well. The fixer also keeps your shadow color in place all day without smudging.

15.  To color and hold your hair: Hair styling foam comes in all hair tints now. Combing them through after shampooing will lightly tint your hair, adding body and shine. You can use foam with any styling method — soft sets, blow drying, heat styling or finger drying. These color-enhancing foams rinse out with one shampoo and do not stain hands or clothing.

16.  To remove a greenish cast from your hair after swimming in a chlorine pool: Use a non-peroxide strawberry henna rinse after shampooing. Your hair will not turn orange; the henna tint will merely neutralize the green.

17.  To freshen up fast: Carry pre-moistened, medicated cleansing pads with you for refreshing hot sticky skin. These are effective in removing perspiration, oil and grime without leaving your skin too dry.

18.  To cure a hangover: You can minimize the effects of heavy drinking by taking two aspirin and drinking as much water as you can before you go to sleep. Keep a glass of water by your bed to assuage your thirst in the middle of the night. When you wake up, drink plenty of mineral water to flush your system, and take a couple of vitamin C tablets. They will give you the energy you need and help your body to fight any infection you may be vulnerable to.

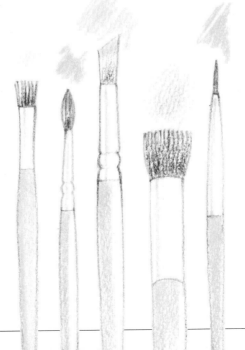

# AGENCIES

CALIFORNIA
**Los Angeles**

Barbizon School
3450 Wilshire Blvd
90010
(School and Agency)
(213) 487-1500

Mary Webb Davis
Agency
515 N. La Cienega
Blvd 90048
(School and Agency)
(213) 652-6850

Caroline Leonetti Ltd
6526 Sunset Blvd
90028
(School and Agency)
(213) 462-2345

Alese Marshall
Enterprises
24050 Vista
Montana, Torrance
90505
(School and Agency)
(213) 378-1223

John Robert Powers
1533 Wilshire Blvd
90017
(School and Agency)
(213) 484-6076

**San Francisco**
Barbizon School of
Modeling
44 Sutter Street
94108
(School and Agency)
(415) 391-4254

Bianca Modeling
260 Stockton Street
94108
(Agency) (415)
495-6700

Brebner Agencies,
Inc.
China Basin Building
No.2
185 Berry Street
94107
(Agency) (415)
495-6700

Cabine International
Models
76 Market Street
(Agency) 94102
(415) 956-2011

John Casablancas/
Elite Models
536 Sutter Street
94102
(Agency)
(415) 433-5483

Demeter & Reed Ltd
70 Zoe Street 94107
(Agency)
(415) 777-1327

Grimme Agency
207 Powell Street
94108
(Agency)
(415) 392-9175

John Robert Powers
28 Geary Street
94108
(School and Agency)
(415) 362-8260

Sabina Models
278 Post Street
94108
(Agency)
(415) 781-6420

Scott Model Agency
760 Market Street
94102
(Agency)
(415) 956-3666

Taaje Models
639 Masson Street
94108  (Agency)
(415) 775-3511

Thibadeau Model
Agency
2229 Market Street
94114
(Agency)
(415) 864-8155

**ILLINOIS**
**Chicago**
Marrise Davidson
and Assoc.
230 N. Michigan
60601
(Agency) (312)
782-4480

ETA Creative Arts
Foundation
7558 S. Chicago
Avenue 60619
(Agency) (312)
752-3955

Shirley Hamilton,
Inc.
620 N. Michigan
Avenue 60611
(Agency)
(312) 644-0300
Cleo Johnson's
School
8445 S. Cottage
Grove Ave. 60619
(School and Agency)
(312) 488-9410

David and Lee
Models
70 W. Hubbard
60610
(Agency)
(312) 661-0500

Playboy Models, Inc
919 N. Michigan
Ave 60611
(Agency)
(312) 664-9024

**MASSACHUSETTS**
**Boston**

Agency for Models
108-A Appleton St.
02116  (Agency)
(617) 267-4211

Bianca Models & Talent
50 Milk St. 02109
(School and Agency)
(617) 426-8371

The Boston Agency
163 Marlboro St. 02116
(Agency)
(617) 247-0200

Cameo Models
392 Boylston St. 02116
(Agency)
(617) 536-6004

Copley 7 Models
29 Newbury St. 02116
(Agency)
(617) 267-4444

Hart Model Agency
137 Newbury St. 02116
(Agency)
(617) 262-1740

The Model Shoppe
176 Newbury St. 02116
(Agency)
(617) 266-6939

Models Group
129 Newbury St 02116
(Agency)
(617) 536-1900

Network Models and Talent
376 Boylston St. 02116 (Agency)
(617) 267-5777

# NEW YORK STATE
## New York City

The Agency Models
9 W 29 Street 10001
(Agency)
(212) 889-8300

The Barbizon
3 E 54 Street 10022
(School and Agency)
(212) 371-4300

Big Beauties
159 Madison Avenue 10016 (Agency)
(212) 685-1270

Sue Charney Models
641 Lexington Ave. 10022
(Agency)
(212) 751-3005

Click
881 Seventh Ave 10019
(Agency)
(212) 245-4306

Grace Del Marco
213 W 53 St 10019
(Agency)
(212) 586-2654

Elite Model Management
110 E. 58 St 10022
(Agency)
(212) 935-4500

Ford Model Agency
344 E. 59 St. 10022
(Agency)
(212) 753-6500

Foster-Fell Agency
26 W. 38 St. 10018
(Agency)
(212) 944-8520

International Model Agency
232 Madison Ave. 10016
(Agency)
(212) 689-5236

Kay Model Agency
111 E. 61 St 10021
(Agency)
(212) 308-9560

Kiki Models
654 Madison Ave. 10021
(Agency)
(212) 888-7111

Legends Model Agency
30 East 34 St., Suite 1600 10016

L'Image Model Management
667 Madison Ave. 10021
(Agency)
(212) 758-6411

Mannequin Models
730 Fifth Avenue 10019
(Agency)
(212) 586-7716

Perkins Models
213 W. 53 St. 10019
(Agency)
(212) 582-9511

Gilla Roos
527 Madison Ave. 10022
(Agency)
(212) 758-5480

Stewart Models
215 E. 81 St. 10028
(Agency)
(212) 249-5540

Wilhelmina Model Agency
9 East 37 Street 10016
(Agency)
(212) 532-6800

Zoli
146 East 56 Street 10022
(Agency)
(212) 758-5959

# FLORIDA
## Miami

All Star Productions Model Agency
Miami International Merchandise Mart
777 NW 72nd Avenue 33126
(Agency)
(305) 261-1343

American Entertainment Mngt. Corp.
1893 NE 164 St., North Miami Beach 33162 (Agency)
(305) 944-0165

Charmette Modeling
Agency
500 Deer Run Drive,
Miami Springs
33166 (Agency)
(305) 871-8253

## GEORGIA
### Atlanta

Atlanta Models and
Talent
3030 Peachtree Rd.
NE 50309 (Agency)
(404) 261-9627

Chez Agency
922 W. Peachtree
St. 30309
(Agency)
(404) 588-1215

Len Chris Ann
School of Modeling
789 Roswell Street
Marietta 30060
(Agency)
(404) 427-4102

Models Touch
2945 Stone Hogan
Rd. Cont. 30311
(Agency)
(404) 346-1210

The Seitz Modeling
Agency
130 Wieuca Rd.
30342
(Agency) (404)
257-9270

The Talent Shop
3379 Peachtree Rd
30326
(Agency)
(404) 261-0770

## MICHIGAN
### Detroit

Affiliated Models
28860 Southfield Rd
Southfield 48076
(Agency)
(313) 559-3110

Maxine Powell
2097 W. Grand
Blvd. 48208
(School)
(313) 897-1520

Patricia Stevens
School
1900 W. Big
Beaver Rd
Troy 48084
(School)
(313) 643-1900

## OHIO
### Cleveland

David Lee Modeling
Agency
The Chesterfield
Bldg. 1801 E 12 St
44114
(Agency)
(216) 522-1300

Dorian Leigh
Modeling Agency
1375 Euclid Ave.
Suite 404 44115
(Agency)
(216) 799-1188

Perfect Images
1258 Euclid Ave.
44115
(Agency)
(216) 696-8589

John Robert Powers
1290 Euclid Ave.
44115
(Agency)
(216) 696-3066

## PENNSYLVANIA
### Philadelphia

Fashion Models
Guild
24 W. Chelten Ave
19144
(Agency)
(215) 844-8872

Kingsley Six Agency
1315 Walnut Street
19107
(Agency)
(215) 546-5919

Models Guild of
Philadelphia
1512 Spruce St.
19102
(Agency)
(215) 735-5606

Studio Guild Agency
1126 Walnut 10107
(Agency)
(215) 925-2101

### Pittsburgh

Walter Brown
Associates
1300 Clark Building
15222
(Agency)
(412) 391-8788

The Wheeler School
P.O. Box 2559 15230
(School and Agency)
(412) 288-4060

## TEXAS
### Dallas

About Face
2524 Converse
75207
(Agency)
(214) 634-0354

Barbizon Agency
12700 Hillcrest
75230
(School and Agency)
(214) 980-7477

Blair-Casablancas
3000 Carlisle 75204
(Agency)
(214) 761-9001

Dallas-Julie Wray
Agency
4330 N. Central
Expwy. 75206
(Agency)
(214) 522-2030

Kim Dawson
Agency
1643 Apparel Mart
75258
(Agency)
(214) 638-2414

The Gill Group
6309 N. O'Conner,
Irving 75039
(Agency)
(214) 869-0666

The Norton Agency
3023 Routh St.
75201
(Agency)
(214) 749-0900

## Houston

Aaron Che Modeling
Agency
P.O. Box 56789
(Agency)
(713) 784-5811

Barbizon
3201 Kirby Dr.
77098
(School and Agency)
(713) 526-6311

d'Lyn Agency
3300 Chimney Rock
77056
(Agency)
(713) 781-5216

Gerri Halpin Agency
911 Kipling 77006
(Agency)
(713) 526-5747

The Holland Group
2209 McArthur
77030
(Agency)
(713) 664-7700

The Mad Hatter
Agency
7249 Ashcroft,
Building B 77081
(Agency)
(713) 995-9090

Intermedia Agency,
Inc
2323 S. Voss, Suite
610 77057
(Agency)
(713) 789-3993

Mayo Hills Actors
and Models of
Houston
7676 Woodway,
Suite 276 77063
(Agency)
(713) 789-4973

Models Unlimited
5420 Stonington
77040
(Agency)
(713) 462-3414

Beverly Wright
Models
4100 Westheimer,
Suite 151 77027
(School and Agency)
(713) 961-0534

Sherry Young
Agency
6420 Hillcroft, Suite
319 77081
(Agency)
(713) 981-9236

## Model Agencies in the United Kingdom

### London

Askew Team
65 New Bond Street,
W1
(01) 493 0631

Bookings
Suite 18/21
12/13 Henrietta
Street, WC2
(01) 836 3821

Count 8
35 Ivor Place, NW1
(01) 723 0314

Crawfords
13 Archer Street, W1
(01) 734 5880

Freddie's
2 Lowndes Street,
SW1
(01) 235 8778

Gavin Robinson
30 Old Bond Street,
W1   (01) 629 5231

Geoff Wootten
51 Brittannia Road,
SW6
(01) 736 0191

Image
81 Wimpole Street,
W1
(01) 935 9021

International
2 Hinde Street, W1
(01) 486 3312

Julia Hunt
124 Gloucester Road,
SW7
(01) 370 1462

Laraine Ashton
6 Cambridge Gate,
NW1
(01) 486 8011

Models One
200 Fulham Road,
SW10
(01) 351 1195

Myrtle Winstone
39 & 41 Sussex Place,
W2
(01) 723 1151

Nevs
36 Walpole Street,
SW3
(01) 730 0615

Penny Personal
11 Addison Avenue,
W11
(01) 602 0021

Premier
69 New Bond Street,
W1
(01) 493 5286

Samantha Bond
241 King's Road,
SW3
(01) 352 3767

Sarah Cape
223a Portobello Road,
W11
(01) 229 1436

# GLOSSARY

**ADVERTISING**  This word encompasses both print and television commercial advertisements for specific products. An *ad* or *advertisement* refers to still photography product promotions.

**ART DIRECTOR**  An art director is one of the people with whom a model works. Art directors design the setting and style of the photographs, editorial spreads, or television commercials. They are usually present during the shoot to 'direct' the photographer, stylist and model(s).

**BEAUTY SHOT**  A full face photograph, such as those on fashion magazine covers. Many advertisers use beauty shots for promoting products such as contact lenses, cosmetics and jewellery.

**BOOK**  A model's portfolio of amateur and/or professional photographs of herself. 'Book' is also used as a verb which means the decision of a client to hire a particular model for a session.

**BOOKING**  Each assignment that a model gets is called a booking.

**BOOKING OUT**  When a model informs her agent that she will not be available for work for a specific number of days in the future. Models are expected to book out at least two weeks in advance.

**CATWALK**  A catwalk is the raised platform that models walk down during fashion shows. The word is also used to describe a fashion show model, as in, 'She's an experienced catwalk talent, she's done all the collection shows this spring.' A catwalk model is also called a *mannequin*.

**CLIENT**  Any person or business that hires a model for a fee, such as a fashion editor of a magazine or a clothing designer.

**COMMISSION**  Modeling agencies usually deduct a 10 per cent commission from a model's earnings.

**COMPOSITE**

A card: 8 x 10in (20 x 25cm) print or brochure printed with a model' photographs, measurements and show business union memberships. Agencies mail composites to clients, and models carry them in their books for presentation.

**CONTACT SHEET (also called CONTACTS)**

A print of all the exposures from a roll, or rolls, or film. Clients and photographers such as hand modeling photographs that a that will be used in print. A model studies contacts to decide which photos she wants as test shots for her book.

**COUTURE (also called HAUTE COUTURE)**

From the French, meaning high fashion, custom designed apparel for women. The first house of haute couture was started in Paris in 1858 by Charles Frederick Worth.

**CREDITS**

The jobs that a model has been paid for, such as hand modelling photographs that a model does for a glove manufacturer, or a string of commercials a model has appeared in.

**DAY RATE**

The fee that a model earns for an all-day single booking. A model also has a basic hourly rate.

**EDITORIAL PRINT WORK**

This is photography that uses models to illustrate fashions and cosmetics for magazines and newspapers; these photos often accompany articles.

**FASHION ILLUSTRATOR**

An artist who draws clothing and fashion accessories for advertising and editorial print work, as well as for catalogs and clothing manufacturers.

**FORMAL MODELING**

This refers to fashion shows that are presented in a stylized, timed format. Formal modeling is a collaborative effort, whereas informal modeling allows models to converse with the public and move independently through department stores, boutiques or restaurant tea rooms.

**GO-SEE**

An interview between model and client that is arranged by the agency to see if the client will book the model for future jobs. A model receives no payment for go-sees; in fact months of go-sees may pass before a model gets her first bookings.

| HEADSHEET | A mailer. catalog, or bound book of photographs and vital statistics of every model represented by an agency. Periodically updated to showcase the models' most recent shots, it is called a headsheet because most of the photos in it are head shots. Headsheets are mailed to past, present and prospective clients. |
|---|---|
| HIGH FASHION | An adjective used in modeling to describe the type of models whose looks are appropriate for couture print and catwalk work. A high fashion model must be at least 5ft 8in (1.73m), very slender, and with well-defined bone structure. |
| LOCATION | A photo session that takes place anywhere except in a photographer's studio. |
| MANNEQUIN | This means both life-sized models of the human figure and live fashion models who pose on the catwalk or in a designer's showroom. |
| PRINT | The final result of a photography session, which is usually an 8 x 10in (20 x 25cm) photograph. |
| PRINT WORK | This term is applied to all bookings that involve still photography, such as catalog, newspaper, magazine and advertising jobs. |
| RELEASE FORM | Every time a client books a model, there is a contractual agreement that must be honored on both sides. A standard printed form, called a model release form, details the terms of their agreement and defines the use of the photographs that will result from the booking. The signature of client and model on the release makes it official. See also *Work Voucher*. |
| RESHOOT | If a client cannot use the results of a print or television commercial booking, he or she will rehire the model to reshoot, paying her the same wages she received for the first booking. |
| RESIDUALS | When a model appears in a television commercial, she earns wages for the time spent making it, plus future (residual) payments that are determined by the |

services she provided in the production and the amount of airtime the commercial is given. Specific working conditions can also affect the pay scale of your residual paychecks.

SHOT
A particular photograph, exposure, slide or frame of film on a contact sheet.

SHOOT
When used as a verb, 'to shoot' is synonymous with taking photographs. As a noun, the word shoot means the entire process of a photo session, and is often used interchangeably with 'booking'.

SPREAD
A feature of one or more photographs appearing in a magazine or newspaper.

STYLIST
A stylist is the production manager of every session, as he or she works with clients and photographers on selecting the props, accessories and clothes for the shoot. The stylist is the person who also obtains these items and then 'styles' them into a scene which the client and photographer can agree to photograph.

TEARSHEETS
These are print clippings from magazines or newspapers that a model puts in her portfolio as soon as they are published.

TEST
(TEST SHOOT)
When a model and photographer agree to do a session for the purpose of producing professional quality photographs of the model for her book. No payment is involved; testing can benefit both parties if the resulting photographs are a success.

TRADE
The different members of the business network that the modeling industry deals with. For example, advertising agency personnel, modeling agency staffers, clients, photographers, stylists, makeup artists, designers, manufacturers and buyers are all in the trade.

WORK
VOUCHER
These are modeling agency work records that are given to models to take to bookings. The client's signature on the work voucher certifies that the booking took place. Agency, client and model all receive a carbon copy of the voucher. Agencies use them to determine the model's wages and to bill the clients.

# INDEX

Quarto would like to thank the following for pictures:

| | |
|---|---|
| Chris Thomson | 14, 15, 16, 17, 18, 19, 20, 24, 27, 34, 37, 38, 39, 41, 42, 43, 44, 45, 48, 49, 53, 55, 56, 57, 58, 61, 62, 63, 64, 65, 66/7, 68, 69, 72, 75, 76, 77, 78, 79, 80, 81, 85(t), 86, 87, 88, 89, 90, 91, 119, 120, 122/123, 127, 128, 137, 138/139, 141, 142, 152/153, 154/155, 156/157, 158/159 |
| Cyndy Warwick | 36, 68 (b), 148, 161, 167 |
| Camera Press | 92, 93, 104, 105, 106, 107, 110, 111 |
| Pineapple Dance Studio, Covent Garden, London | 12/13, 85 (b) |
| Tony Stone Worldwide | 21, 22, 23 |
| Laura Ashley | 113, 130, 131 |
| John Heseltine | 95, 96, 97 |
| Wallis Fashions — clothes from 1984 winter collection | 90 (t), 114, 115 |
| Paul Webster — © Marshall Cavendish | 30/31 |
| Hong Kong Tourist Authority | 162/163 |
| Vidal Sassoon, hair by | 70/71 |
| Illustration Terry Evans | 26, 46, 47, 50, 51, 52, 53, 54, 59, 60, 100, 103 |
| John Galliano | 99 |
| Greg Myler | 98 |
| Key | (t) top, (b) bottom |